Strategic Debriefing for Advanced Simulation

Giorgio Capogna • Pier Luigi Ingrassia
Emanuele Capogna • Michela Bernardini
Elisa Valteroni • Giada Pietrabissa
Giorgio Nardone

Strategic Debriefing for Advanced Simulation

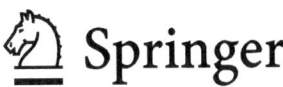

Giorgio Capogna
EESOA Simulation Centre
ROMA, Roma, Italy

Emanuele Capogna
EESOA Simulation Centre
Roma, Italy

Elisa Valteroni
Strategic Therapy Centre
Arezzo,
Italy

Giorgio Nardone
Strategic Therapy Centre
Arezzo, Italy

Pier Luigi Ingrassia
CeSi Simulation Centre
Lugano, Switzerland

Michela Bernardini
SIMNOVA Simulation Centre
Novara, Italy

Giada Pietrabissa
Faculty of Psychology
Catholic University of the Sacred Heart
Milano, Italy

ISBN 978-3-031-06103-5   ISBN 978-3-031-06104-2   (eBook)
https://doi.org/10.1007/978-3-031-06104-2

Contents

1   What You Need to Know Before You Start   1
1.1   Error in Medicine: From Fault to Resource   1
    1.1.1   Error Classification   3
    1.1.2   Working with Error in Simulation for Patient Safety   5
    1.1.3   The Human Factor: Training Non-technical Skills
            with CRM   8
1.2   Adult Learning in Simulation   14
    1.2.1   Experiential Learning: The Kolb Cycle   16
    1.2.2   Learning from the Experience of the Other:
            Mirror Neurons   18
    1.2.3   Protected Learning and Psychological Safety   20
1.3   Training Methods: From Frontal Lesson to Simulation.   21
1.4   Elements and Characteristics of Communication   23
References.   25

2   Essentials of Debriefing   27
2.1   Definition of Debriefing.   27
2.2   Purpose of Debriefing and Learning Objectives   28
2.3   Debriefing Participants.   29
2.4   When, Where, and How Long to Debrief   30
2.5   Qualities of the Debriefer.   31
2.6   Structure of the Debriefing.   32
2.7   Communication Methods Used in Debriefing   34
    2.7.1   Feedback (Directive, Peer, and Self-feedback)   34
    2.7.2   Plus/Delta.   35
    2.7.3   Assertion-Investigation   36
2.8   Debriefing and Structural Deficits in the Working
    Environment.   36
2.9   The Co-debriefing   37
2.10 Concluding Remarks   38
References.   39

3   Effective Communication for Strategic Change 43
  3.1   Introduction 43
  3.2   Knowing to See by Learning How to Act: Theory Informing
         the Brief Strategic Approach 45
  3.3   The Structure of the Strategic Dialogue 46
         3.3.1   Use of the Strategic Questioning 48
         3.3.2   Reframing and Paraphrases 50
         3.3.3   Evoking Sensation 50
         3.3.4   Summarize to Redefine 51
  3.4   Prescription as an Outcome 51
  3.5   Conclusion 52
  References 52

4   Strategic Debriefing: A Corrective Emotional Experience 55
  4.1   Emotions and Simulation 56
  4.2   How to Help Learners Deal with the Emotions Felt During the
         Scenario 58
  4.3   Descriptive Phase 59
  4.4   Analytical Phase 60
  4.5   Application Phase 63
  4.6   General Considerations 64
  4.7   Psychotraps and Their Use in Simulation 64
         4.7.1   The Deception of Expectations 65
         4.7.2   The Illusion of Ultimate Knowledge 66
         4.7.3   The Myth of Perfect Reasoning 67
         4.7.4   I Felt It, Then Is 67
         4.7.5   Consistency at All Costs 67
         4.7.6   Overestimate/Underestimate 68
  References 68

5   Strategic Debriefing in Practice 69
  5.1   Briefing Before the Scenario 70
  5.2   What to Do During the Scenario 71
  5.3   Reaction and *De-roling* Phase 75
         5.3.1   In Basic Debriefing 76
         5.3.2   In Strategic Debriefing 77
  5.4   How to Start Debriefing: The Introduction to the Method 78
  5.5   Descriptive Phase 79
         5.5.1   In Basic Debriefing 79
         5.5.2   In Strategic Debriefing 80
  5.6   The Analytical Phase 81
         5.6.1   In Basic Debriefing 83
         5.6.2   In Strategic Debriefing 87

5.7   The Application Phase   91
     5.7.1   In Basic Debriefing   91
     5.7.2   In Strategic Debriefing.   92
5.8   The Difficult Debriefing.   94
5.9   How to Evaluate the Debriefing.   97
References.   101

Appendixes.   103

1

Errare humanum est/To err is human

Augustine of Hippo

1.1 Error in Medicine: From Fault to Resource

You are drinking your coffee comfortably seated on your sofa, and you realize that it tastes disgusting: there is salt! Maybe a member of your family has inadvertently swapped salt with sugar, or they were put in similar jars, or maybe the label of one of the two has come off, or maybe this morning you were still so sleepy that you could not distinguish the two jars. The fact is that your coffee is salty and really undrinkable. "Who did this?" It is inherent in our culture and our daily way of thinking to ponder the causes of an event to find out who the culprit is.

This question is the result of a "culture of error" that guides us in our search for the person responsible, the person who made the mistake, and the person who put salt in the coffee.

In its common sense, the word error means a deviation from a linear path; in fact, it derives from the Latin *error/oris* which means "to wander, to err." This definition leads to a deviation from the right path and indicates an abnormal or even pathological behavior.

However, there are many inventions and discoveries that came about not only through creative intuition but also through mistakes, such as penicillin, post-its, mirror neurons, etc.

Einstein said that "we can't expect things to change if we keep doing the same things" and that "crisis is the greatest blessing for people and nations, because crisis brings progress [...] it is in crisis that inventiveness, discoveries and great strategies arise."

In healthcare, there is not always this positive conception of error, as medical error can cause harm to the patient.

Often, the responsibility is attributed to the individual professional who finds himself to be the final link in a chain of factors that have contributed to the occurrence of harm to the patient, ignoring the organizational and systemic dimension in which the individual was operating.

© The Author(s), under exclusive license to Springer Nature
Switzerland AG 2022
G. Capogna et al., *Strategic Debriefing for Advanced Simulation*,
https://doi.org/10.1007/978-3-031-06104-2_1

According to this person-based approach, if something goes wrong, it is solely the fault of the person who made the material error. He did not have the necessary knowledge, was not careful enough, or did not do his best. Mistakes are attributed to lack of knowledge, lack of attention, and lack of motivation or negligence, and the result is a culture of blaming, scolding, and mortifying.

According to this perspective, mistakes are avoided by improving knowledge (e.g., with better training) and increasing motivation with warnings ("be more careful next time," "if you concentrate well, you won't make mistakes again") or with threats of disciplinary procedures.

This approach is functional for a healthcare institution that wants to maintain a blameless public image. Instead of looking for institutional responsibility internally, it is easier and cheaper to focus on the individuals who made mistakes. This person-based approach, however, misses the opportunity to improve patient safety by correcting healthcare organizations, because it isolates dangerous actions from their context in the system. Far from being random, incidents tend to fit into recurring patterns. A similar set of circumstances can result in similar errors, regardless of the healthcare personnel involved. This explains why error is not the monopoly of an unlucky few: analysis of accidents in other high-risk technological environments (e.g., civil aviation, nuclear facilities, space exploration) shows that it is often "the best people who make the worst mistakes" [1]. This happens because sometimes, with more experience, people tend to become complacent, or simply because the most difficult tasks are assigned to the most experienced people.

It is therefore reductive to attribute error to the individual, the ultimate executor of a series of actions for which he or she is not necessarily primarily responsible. We must, instead, consider each professional within a system that is composed of the organization, culture, tools, procedures, devices, supervision, human resource management, and communication between those present.

When the focus shifts from the individual person to the processes, you have a "systems approach."

According to this view, instead of looking for a single determining action and, therefore, a single responsible person as being responsible for the incident, all levels of the organization are carefully examined, looking for the factors that contributed to that error. The basic premise in the systems approach is that human beings are fallible and that errors must be anticipated, even in the best organizations.

For example, when an adverse event happens, and a patient is harmed, the main issue will not be who made a mistake, but rather why and how the system's defenses failed and what were the upstream systemic factors that contributed to the incident. Focusing on the system and its weaknesses provides valuable information for further improvement. So, instead of asking who is to blame, we should ask, "What exactly went wrong? How many different types of failure occurred? Is it possible to do a temporal reconstruction of key events? Why did things go wrong? What psychological mechanisms contributed to the development of the accident? How did the various organizational and human factors interact to cause the accident?"

Therefore, mistakes should not be hidden but considered a resource: what is important is not making a mistake in itself but what we do with that mistake, that is, how we deal with it.

From the point of view of error as a resource, simulation plays a fundamental role in that it is a useful and "painless" means of replicating the error in a protected environment that first and foremost guarantees the safety of the patient and the learner.

In addition, what is essential in simulation is the "psychological protection" of their learners who, not feeling "guilty and judged," will not run the risk of losing their positive self-image, and denying the error or hiding it instead of sharing it.

For these reasons, in the post-simulation debriefing, it is important to create a climate of listening and non-judgmental acceptance that makes learners feel free to express themselves without fear of being attacked or criticized, to encourage a process of growth and evolution, starting from their mistakes, which can be taken as an integral part of their lives and their professional career.

The way in which the debriefer approaches the error will condition the way we conduct the debriefing: having a non-judgmental attitude and behavior toward our learners will depend, above all, on the vision that we ourselves have, both of our own errors and of the errors of others. For this reason, it is important to be aware of our attitude and of the fallout in terms of learning of our learners.

1.1.1 Error Classification

When an adverse event occurs and a patient is harmed, one should speak of an organizational accident rather than of human error. The main issue to be addressed is not who made the mistake, but why and how the system's defenses failed, i.e., what were the systemic factors upstream that contributed to the incident.

In the study of factors that influence the efficiency and reliability of performance at work, the most widely used model of reference is the skill-rule-knowledge postulated by Rasmussen [2] who proposes a classification of human behavior that responds to a critical situation based on the degree of familiarity with similar situations.

Rasmussen's model indicates three different categories of error-related behavior, based on experience and familiarity: *skill-based behavior*, *rule-based behavior*, and *knowledge-based behavior*.

The three levels of performance correspond to different levels of familiarity with the environment or task, as experience and familiarity with a situation allow the practitioner to use his/her "skills, rules and knowledge."

Skill-based behavior: literally means routine behavior based on learned skills. This is the level of skills, the abilities that refer to all those automatisms acquired through exercise. Walking, driving, cycling, and tying our shoes are our daily *skill-based behaviors*: routine actions and behaviors that we carry out without consciously thinking about them and without having a conscious memory of having done them because the cognitive effort required is very low and reasoning is unconscious.

The utmost familiarity with these actions leads us to make unintentional mistakes and oversights, i.e., actions performed differently from what was planned.

In rule-based behavior, usual problems are addressed whose solutions are given by the simple application of rules. For example, the caregiver has all the algorithms and procedures to perform known tasks; he only has to recognize the situation and apply the appropriate procedure to perform the task and solve the problem. Errors at this level may be due to a misapplied rule, applying the wrong rule well, or not applying a rule at all, such as a doctor not recognizing that a flu fever may be meningitis and therefore not applying the appropriate procedure.

In knowledge-based behavior, the behavior is knowledge-based and aimed at solving problems in the presence of situations that are not habitual and not very familiar.

The errors referred to in this behavior are those linked to partial, incorrect knowledge or errors in the assessment of the situation and for which a specific procedure has never been defined.

Based on the model proposed by Rasmussen, three different types of errors have been identified: *slip*, *lapse*, and *mistake*. The first two are execution errors, and the third is a scheduling error.

The *slip error* is an error of execution that occurs at the skill level; it is given by the unintentional inability to complete the task; it concerns a lack in the execution of an action. A *slip* error is a "slip," such as grabbing the television remote control in the act of answering a call when the cell phone rings. They are such obvious and automatic actions that require minimal cognitive effort and can occur due to distraction or perhaps because we are overthinking. The intention was good, to answer the phone, but the execution was wrong, gripping the remote control like a handset.

Another example of a *slip* is inadvertently selecting the wrong energy level on your defibrillator or prescribing a different medication than you had in mind because you got distracted.

Lapses are errors of execution caused by a memory deficit; they occur when some important steps in a sequence of actions are omitted, due to environmental distractions or to forgetfulness or carelessness. The cause of the occurrence of *lapses* is to be attributed to the automatic memorization of procedures learned with repeated practice, and that can also be carried out in an unconscious way. The *lapses* are involuntary forgetfulness, such as sometimes forgetting the slice of bread in the toaster and remembering only when you are aware of an unpleasant smell of burning. In this category are classified all those actions performed differently than planned, that is, the operator knows how he should perform a task, but does not do it, or inadvertently performs it incorrectly.

Mistakes are errors due to a deficient plan of action despite the actions being implemented as they were planned. They can be of two types: *rule-based* and *knowledge-based*. The first are errors due to the choice of the wrong rule because of a misperception of the situation; the second are errors due to lack of knowledge or its incorrect application. The negative result of the action lies in the erroneous knowledge that led to it. The error based on knowledge is caused by a wrong attempt to solve a situation that one knows little about, as if a cardiologist was asked to take care of a patient with oncological problems, or a rather rare pathology that he does not know.

This type of error is inherent in the limited rationality or otherwise the difficulty of giving answers to problems that present a wide range of possible choices [3].

In summary, if in the *skill-based* activities the skill consists in carrying out the task without necessarily having to know the reasons, since they are automatic and elementary activities, in the *rule-based* or *knowledge-based* activities, the operator needs to possess all the knowledge and motivations that underlie the task to be able to perform it properly.

According to the definition of Reason, an aviation psychologist, we speak of error in all those occasions in which a planned sequence of physical or mental activities does not reach its goal, and this is not because someone has intervened to prevent the achievement of that goal but because the dynamics involved are many and complex.

1.1.2   Working with Error in Simulation for Patient Safety

Not all the mistakes we make result in harm or an accident; in fact most of our mistakes have no consequences whatsoever. The errors that we have classified as *slips*, *lapses*, and *mistakes* are active errors because they are visible, they cause accidents in a direct way and have immediate consequences, and they occur when our actions precede an accident, a damage.

However, there are also latent conditions that can remain hidden in the system for a long time, but when they intercept an unsafe action of ours, they turn into an error.

Remember our coffee with salt? Having the same cans for sugar and salt is the latent condition in the system that encourages the active error of swapping salt for sugar to occur.

An incident makes evident those latent errors that were present in the system itself but had not yet manifested themselves. In this regard, Reason [4] introduced the "Swiss cheese" model (Fig. 1.1), in which the cheese slices would represent the barriers and defenses put in place by the organization to intercept the possible trajectory of an error. If the trajectory intercepts all the holes in the cheese that have simultaneously aligned, i.e., the flaws in the system, an incident occurs; if, on the other hand, it encounters a defensive barrier (i.e., the cheese slices with the misaligned holes), the error is intercepted and does not cause negative outcomes.

For an accident to occur, our action must penetrate different layers (different slices of cheese), and each layer is a defensive and protective barrier of the system, which may be deficient, as in the case of lack of supervision (such as not having made a checklist of the equipment in the truck), organizational deficiencies (such as the presence of excessive loads of work, timetables, and shift patterns), unsafe acts (exchange of vials), and the pre-conditions for unsafe acts (tiredness, personal

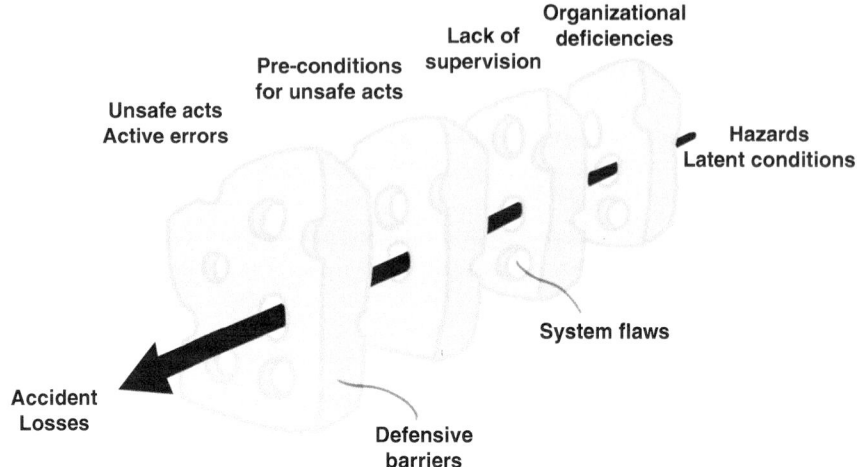

Fig. 1.1 Model of Reason

reasons). If the defensive barriers fail, the holes in the Swiss cheese line up, and the mistake can turn into an accident.

The individual-error approach places all the responsibility on the last piece of cheese, that is, the frontline operator, while the system approach assesses the presence or absence of the other upstream protective barriers that prevent the error committed by the individual from generating an accident.

Basically, according to this theory, errors that threaten safety may be made by the person treating the patient at that moment, or they may be the result of decisions already made, in times and places much more distant than the moment of the error. These errors remain latent within the system and may remain so for a very long time, until they contribute to an undesirable event. In essence, active errors and latent conditions differ in the location/level of an organization in which they occur and the amount of time that passes before they reveal an adverse effect on safety.

Active errors are the most visible and cause adverse events or accidents in a direct way, thus causing immediate consequences. Swapping vials and injecting the wrong medication are examples of active errors. Precisely because active errors are easily identified, they become the subject of thorough investigations and often lead to sanctions of the "individual responsible."

However, safety-critical decisions can also be made by people on the other side of the organization, "not on the frontline." Such decisions are made far from the patient, both in terms of time and physical distance, and yet, they themselves have a potential negative effect on the patient, causing latent errors. These decisions are made at every level of the organization: decisions at the highest level, as well as simple administrative acts, can create conditions that facilitate workplace accidents. Latent conditions are hidden within the organization, in structures (e.g., the architectural design of an intensive care unit, electromedical equipment, computer programs), and in processes (e.g., operating procedures, internal guidelines, personnel selection, qualification procedures, human resource management). In every complex system, at any given time, there is a certain amount of hidden latent conditions. Years or even decades may pass before these decisions have consequences for a patient. Until that day, no one would classify them as "errors" even though there is sufficient evidence that latent conditions pose the greatest threat to the safety of a system. Healthcare organizations are particularly vulnerable to latent errors because they must establish resources for two different goals, productivity and safety, which often come into conflict.

An example of a latent error might be a management decision to assign only one physician per operating room, without having a supervising anesthesiologist free to help less experienced staff: this working condition represents a latent condition for possible errors that can trigger a critical situation.

Good teamwork is also an essential element in preventing errors and accidents in medicine. There is a clear relationship between good teamwork and effective performance in the high-risk healthcare environment [5].

One of the most important causes of poor organization and teamwork is the lack of a shared understanding of the importance of this issue, and the actions necessary for good teamwork. As a result, conflicts between team members and a breakdown in communication can undermine collaboration and lead to under- or misuse of available resources and the emergence of new problems. In addition, team members may not share the same assessment of the situation and may be reluctant to question the actions of other participants, even when there are serious concerns about the appropriateness of a diagnosis or treatment.

Safety is therefore a complex concept and difficult to explain, as it seems to be invisible. Much like "health," the word "security" suffers from an instability of understanding. Much more is known "about its temporary absence than about its stable presence" [6].

Just as health is not merely the absence of disease, so safety is not merely the absence of accidents or errors, nor is it a static feature of the system, as Weick [7] states, but a "dynamic non-event," that is, a dynamic absence of critical events, which must be maintained by individuals and teams.

Security is therefore a dynamic task, requiring a series of proactive measures to achieve stable results, considering that the best solution to a problem is not a person but a system response.

Our healthcare organizations are often oriented toward preventing errors rather than promoting safety. When we think about preventing an error, we talk about reactive safety only after the incident has taken place, but there is also proactive safety that establishes actions to be taken before an incident caused by an error occurs [8].

In the 1990s, there was an important change of view given by the publication of "To Err is human" [9]. In this report, it was shown that the error is dependent on many factors and not only on the attention or memory problems of those who commit it. Since then, the error is no longer and not only considered as a characteristic of the human being, but of all systems that include humans.

In fact, the analysis of many adverse events in healthcare has revealed that many causes of error originate from deficits in non-technical performance, such as communication, teamwork, and situational awareness, rather than from a lack of technical and procedural competence [10].

The inappropriate organization of processes and interventions and the environment in which care is delivered play a much more significant role in causing harm than the error made by the individual. Although error is impossible to eliminate completely, it becomes necessary to create systems that minimize the likelihood of errors while maximizing the probability of intercepting them. If to err is human, then one must make the system as safe as possible.

Training of healthcare personnel is one of the most functional strategies for reducing errors and improving work performance, and should not only focus on technical aspects but also extend to non-technical skills.

Simulation permits the dealing with training aspects related to both technical and non-technical skills, offering the tools to work, according to Rasmussen's behavioral models, on skills, rules, and knowledge.

The learner who participates in a simulation and debriefing session has the opportunity to reflect on his or her actions and independently verify the effectiveness of his or her actions, achieving greater self-awareness.

In this training context, debriefing takes on its highest form of usefulness because it allows access to all those teamwork dynamics that are often the key to solving critical situations that individually would not be solvable.

1.1.3   The Human Factor: Training Non-technical Skills with CRM

It was January 15, 2009, when what the media called "The Miracle on the Hudson" occurred, when airline pilot Chesley "Sully" Burnett, in command of a stalled plane after a bird-strike, made an emergency landing on the Hudson River saving the 155 passengers. After the rescue, he was considered a national hero even though some tried to destroy his career.

We quote this true story, told in a beautiful film starring Tom Hanks (Sully 2016, directed by Clint Eastwood), because it describes when and how the human factor makes a difference: Commander Sully is a fine example of resilience.

The film starts with disciplinary proceedings against the commander and co-pilot of the plane: human error is presumed, because, although the disaster was averted, procedures were not followed and suggestions from the control tower and availability for landing were not accepted.

The question arises: is Sully a hero or an irresponsible one?

In the film, it is clearly shown that it was not "human error," but rather "human factor": it was the ability of man, in this case the great personality and professionalism of Commander Sully, to take the risk of a decision that was not a simple application of rules and customs, but rather the ability to consider all the factors at play in the specific situation and draw the best operational consequences.

When faced with computer and manual simulations that tend to show that the proposed landings would have been possible without damage to the aircraft and people, Sully claims that the human factor should be considered in the reconstruction, that is, those few seconds that it took him to become aware of the situation and decide for the ditching as the only viable alternative. With the addition of those seconds, even the simulations change and show how wise and valuable his choice was.

Sully also adds that this "Hudson miracle," as they called it, was possible because of teamwork, meaning everyone: the co-pilot, the flight crew, the passengers, and the control tower staff.

Human factor "is the study of human potentials, limitations, and behaviors, and the integration of this knowledge into the design phase of the things, places, and work environments in which human beings live and work in order to improve the efficiency, safety, and well-being of people" [11].

The human factor started to be discussed in aeronautics, when they began to study the causes of many air accidents. Scholars have come to argue that accidents were not so much related to the adequacy of professional skills possessed by operators, but to the failure to exercise non-technical skills, for example, communication skills and teamwork. In fact, the technical skills and competences of pilots alone have not been considered sufficient to guarantee the safety of flight operations and to avoid accidents [12].

Non-technical skills (NTS) are involved in the definition of the human factor and are personal and social cognitive skills that integrate with the technical skills of operators and professionals. The most relevant are situational awareness, *decision-making*, teamwork, *leadership*, and, transversally, communication.

NTS are particularly relevant in high-complexity organizations and professions, such as pilots, doctors, hospital staff, and high-risk categories of workers, thus the aviation and healthcare sectors.

Whether we are flying in an airplane or entering an operating room to undergo surgery, we are entrusted to teams of professionals who manage a complex system (operating room or cockpit), perform complex processes, govern high technologies, and manage the human component which is the most important factor for the success of the process of care and safety of patients and passengers.

The aviation industry has identified NTS training as the best way to protect specialists and organizations from mistakes and accidents. In 1981, United Airlines began specific training to make crews aware of the dynamics of human interaction on board and to recognize behaviors found in operational life.

These trainings were called *crew resource management* (CRM), and they constituted and still constitute one of the most effective models of transversal training on work groups, based on the definition of shared mental and behavioral models, on the improvement of safety, and on the training and promotion of non-technical attitudes and behaviors that contribute to the success of a mission through a training method addressed to the totality of the members of the team and not to the single individual.

CRM courses, now successfully tested in aviation, were later transferred to the healthcare field thanks to David Gaba et al. [13], an anesthesiologist and professor at Stanford University, and his collaborators who adapted the aviation model to emergency situations, thus giving birth to *anesthesia crisis resource management* (ACRM).

CRM in the healthcare field maintains the same acronym but with a different meaning; in fact, it stands for *crisis resource management*, where *crisis* can be a sudden crisis of the pathological conditions of a patient, a crisis of *leadership*, and a crisis of communication or of situational awareness in the healthcare team.

"Crisis" is also an unexpected, life-threatening event in which there is a disparity between the resources available and those needed to stabilize the patient's standard vitals.

By "resources" we mean a wide range of tools, personal, psychological, and material to be activated to improve the patient's condition. For example, in a case of copious hemorrhage, the patient can be treated without particular difficulty in the operating room because of the wide availability of professional experience, instrumentation, blood, and fluids. The same patient, in any medical ward, could, on the contrary, represent a critical case in the case of an unexpected event, in the absence of specialized personnel and essential tools for rescue.

In this circumstance, the requirements for the best management of the emergency are the immediate understanding of the situation, its possible evolution, the possibilities of a solution, and the involvement of several actors in the management of the crisis.

The term *crisis resource management* (CRM) refers to all those non-technical skills necessary for effective teamwork in a crisis situation, where high-level performance is the result of the collaboration of all team members.

In the debriefing phase, it is important to know the CRM principles and recall them, if appropriate, as they emphasize the human factors and NTS involved in managing the critical scenario.

The CRM methodology is widely used in simulation and represents the set of general principles for criticality management and error prevention in emergency situations.

Fifteen key points are identified (Fig. 1.2) that have the common goal of coordinating, utilizing, and applying all available resources to optimize safety and outcomes in patient care.

Let's look at the 15 key points of CRM in more detail:

1. Know your environment: this means not only knowing the spaces where you will have to move but also being informed about what materials and medical devices you have at your disposal and how they work. In addition to the materials, it is also necessary to know the human resources, the work group, and other colleagues who may be available in case of need.
2. Anticipation and planning: both are used to reduce the need for improvisation and to maintain control of the situation, eliminating some of the unforeseen events that can hinder care and potentially make it even more hectic, confusing, and stressful. Knowing the consequences of a problem or crisis and sharing this knowledge with team members help others focus on what needs to be done and prioritized. Dividing roles before the patient even comes to the attention of the

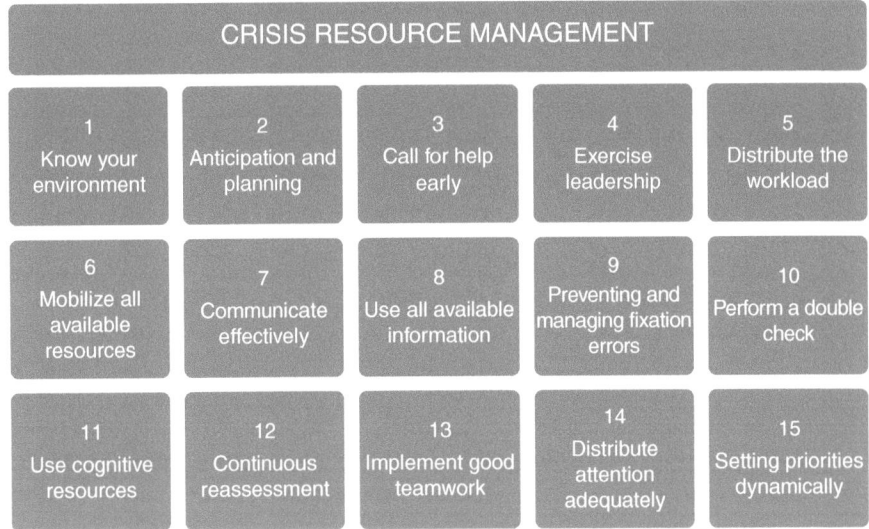

Fig. 1.2   Principles of crisis resource management (CRM)

care team (whether in or out of hospital) minimizes interruptions in agreeing "who does what" and gives the *team leader* more time and focus to devote to the patient.

3. Call for help early: calling for help early is not a sign of weakness, but rather of responsibility toward the patient. Some emergencies are time-dependent and require timely specialist care in order to "rescue" the patient in a short time. In a scenario, simulations can be implemented in a controlled environment, where the patient's problems are known, in order to create situations where outside help is required, and the expectation that help will actually be called can be reinforced. In the case of simulation, errors can be left uncorrected to help learners understand the outcomes of certain actions or non-actions.

4. Exercise *leadership* and team dynamics: being a *leader does* not mean knowing more than others, doing everything alone, and overpowering others or imposing oneself, but coordinating operators in their roles in the intervention through clear and effective communication of provisions. The *leader is* responsible for coordinating the activities of the individuals in a team according to the needs and priorities of a given situation. On the other hand, the team members must also listen to the *leader*, carry out the given instructions, and make sure that the *leader* is informed of any concerns about the course of action. In this way, the *leader* and the team members support each other, and this greatly reduces the levels of anxiety and stress in managing the emergency.

In a simulation and subsequent debriefing, a significant number of leadership issues can be examined such as the *leader*'s perception of what happened, how he or she communicated with the group, the group members' perceptions of *leadership, the leader*'s listening skills, role allocation within the team, and resource management.

5. Distribute the workload: this reduces the physical and emotional overload that can be inevitable for the key figures involved in an emergency. In addition, the distribution of responsibilities and workload prevents the team from operating at different speeds. Understanding which tasks are the responsibility of the individual professional and which can be assigned to others saves energy and resources that can be saved for crucial moments. In some emergency simulations, we assume that the best *leaders* in the various professions or specialties are those who can adequately manage workloads and understand the difficulties of each professional.

6. Mobilize all available resources: limit the workload and allow the team to work in the best possible conditions, reducing stress due to excessive time pressure or the lack of resources deemed essential in the emergency. It is directly related to the knowledge of the environment, since it is necessary for the team to have a thorough knowledge of all the resources that it has available and that it can call upon in case of need (personnel, equipment, materials, etc.).

7. Communicate effectively: Communication is the act of sending and receiving information and orders and making judgements in a clear manner. It is the responsibility of each member of a team to understand what is being said and, in turn, to make themselves understood. Communication should be clear and closed loop and always include *feedback* to facilitate the interlocutors and prevent mistakes and delay in achieving the set goals. Excessively long sentences should not be used, and the interlocutors should speak to each other by name and look each other in the eyes, so as to be sure of having communicated the right thing to the right person. Obstacles to good communication are distractions in the group, hierarchies, or lack of a shared model for dealing with a situation or problem. Noise, interpersonal problems, or *leader* behavior can impair communication or the respondent's willingness to ask for clarification.

8. Use all available information: do not dismiss information that is apparently not relevant to the emergency situation, as sometimes, it is only knowledge of it that can help resolve it. In many emergencies, data may be inaccurate, incomplete, or artifactual, and it is necessary to respond to the data in a way that is appropriate to the actual condition.

9. Preventing and managing fixation errors: fixation errors are generated by a persistent failure to reassess or evaluate further alternatives. Engagement in practices that have little relation to the main problem, or in some manuals, is the most common evidence of this type of error. DeKeyser and Woods [14] describe three main types of fixation errors:

    (a) This and only this: failing to give proper consideration to the rare, but correct alternative because of persistent fixation on a single problem and failing to review diagnosis or future planning, despite evidence that contradicts them (e.g., treating tachycardia instead of major bleeding, etc.).

    (b) Anything but this: excluding a priori the possibility of considering an alternative; inability to act on the main problem. Considerable time is wasted looking for other causes, sometimes to the exclusion of dealing with the main one.

(c) All is well: the problem is not recognized, and consequently, the possibility to act is excluded. Generally reassuring signs or symptoms are used to set aside the more worrisome evidence (e.g., despite anuria and increased lactates, the patient is conscious, so no urgency to treat the patient, etc.). Similarly, data of concern are deleted and considered artifactual, even if they indicate impending deterioration. Equipment problems, alarms, and abnormal data can introduce improper changes in framing.

The awareness of the fixing errors that a CRM course brings to light leads to the establishment of specific rules applicable to every workplace. Care protocols and requests for help, which are mandatory in specific critical circumstances, and an atmosphere in which all staff members feel they can make a valuable contribution, are the ideal conditions for avoiding biased errors.

10. Perform a double check: it consists in the constant verification of one's own work and that of others, thus allowing the operator to work safely, reducing the anxiety of making mistakes, and also decreasing the feeling of pressure from unilateral control.

11. Use cognitive resources, instrumental, and not to draw on all available knowledge resources, such as procedure checklists, memos, manuals, electronic instruments, calculators to calculate dosages, guidelines to consult to confirm a course of action, dedicated applications of the mobile phone with respect to the drugs to be administered, handbooks, etc. This does not diminish the knowledge of the operator (who cannot be omniscient) but also allows you to act with greater confidence and precision. Following the ABC in the case of an uncertain situation is a cognitive modality that everyone has trained to fulfil, but beyond this, in medical practice, intended both as medical training and as workplace, very little has been done to encourage the use of decision support tools.

Since the early days of CRM training in healthcare, cognitive tools have been strongly recommended as decision support.

12. Continuous reassessment: this is used to identify important clinical changes that occur in the emergency situation. This process makes it possible to keep abreast of the most important problems that arise from time to time and that require attention from the entire team. In this way, it is an indispensable working tool for continually reshaping the established intervention plan.

13. Implement good teamwork: it allows for the sharing of anxieties and concerns in order to better manage the emergency situation, as well as to combine all the knowledge coming from different areas of expertise in order to respond in the most complete and appropriate way to the needs of the patient. It should be emphasized that behind every team, there is, first of all, the work of setting up the group, where the individuals who make up the group make available parts of themselves, even giving up something and acquiring other things from the closeness with the others.

14. Distribute attention adequately: concentrating on the most important things is a determining element in emergency management. The operator, while receiving a lot of information, often at the same time, must process it quickly establishing priorities because he cannot perform several procedures at the same time, but only in rapid sequence. This reduces not only the possibility of error but also the stress of operational pressure.
15. Setting priorities dynamically: "What was right before may not be right now and vice versa." Assessing priorities dynamically helps the practitioner not to be left behind by the evolution of the situation and allows him to act accordingly to "what is happening now."

CRM training in healthcare simulation allows for the training in all those non-technical skills necessary for effective teamwork in a crisis situation, where high-level performance is the result of the collaboration of all team members.

In CRM training, we do not teach a technique or a methodology to respond to a crisis, to an emergency, but we try to make every single participant aware of how he/she reacts in that situation, according to the principle that the human factor is yes a limit but above all a resource, as we saw in the example of Commander Sully, in a continuous effort to make a transition from the perspective of error prevention to that of safety promotion [15].

1.2   Adult Learning in Simulation

Do we remember what the last thing we learned was? And what affected the learning?

Let's take the example of learning a new language: it is commonly believed that learning a foreign language as an adult is much more difficult than learning it as a child. We can learn it in a language course, but if we live for a long time in a foreign country immersed in the language to be learned, we will accelerate the learning time. For children, learning is very often associated with play, with fun, a mode that does not always accompany adult learning.

Learning is a relatively long-lasting and stable modification of behavior as a result of an experience, usually repeated several times over time; it is an experiential, trial-and-error process through which our cognitive, emotional, and social behavior changes in response to stimuli in the environment [16].

Learning is a complex process, as it involves our sensations, our emotions, our motivations, our memory, and our unconscious dimension, but also the social, historical, and cultural context within which we live.

In order to learn as an adult, neither intelligence nor rationality is enough, but we also need emotions that act as an anchor for our experiences, allowing us to associate an experience with a lived emotion which, in turn, helps our memory process the information.

Learning as an adult in a Simulation Centre is similar to learning a new language, a new vocabulary, immersed in an experience that makes you adopt new behaviors, previously absent, or makes you more aware of those that were already in place.

All of this is done bearing in mind the emotions that intervene in a learning process and that govern all human relationships, allowing you to open up to the world and enter into a relationship with others. For this reason, becoming familiar with emotions and learning to recognize them essentially means learning to question oneself, to accept oneself, to be open to confrontation, especially in the debriefing phase.

Adult learning is closely related to the dimension of experiencing, of "doing": if we do not experience something, if we do not feel sensations on our skin, we are not in the condition to "learn." The root of learning is experience; all our learning is experiential, and that is why simulation is a pivotal tool for learning [17–19].

Knowles' [20] studies of andragogy, a science that studies adult learning, show that the adult learner is at the center of their own learning process and actively participates throughout.

It derives from the assumption that adults must learn to transform their own life contexts, committing themselves to create an essential link between their own experience and the meaning to be attributed to the experience itself, thus creating, as Dewey et al. [21] claimed, an authentic educational experience.

It follows that simulation training is the first step in the process of acquiring the awareness and knowledge necessary to change working practices.

It is therefore important to define the role of an instructor in a Simulation Center, which relates to adult learners with a high level of professionalism.

The instructor should have the role of a "learning facilitator," a guide, a kind of companion who actively involves people without imposing his own knowledge and ideas. He works on non-technical skills, knows when to step back to leave the scene to the learners, creates a positive and collaborative climate, and stimulates motivation and active participation, making learners aware of the importance of the path to be faced.

The learning facilitator must prepare the environment and set it up for the learner to feel the need and necessity to change independently and thus make themselves responsible for their learning. As Rogers said in support of this "there must be active and personal involvement on the part of the learner for meaningful learning" [22].

It should be remembered that adults learn what they want to learn and what is meaningful to them; they draw on the resources they have already accumulated in the course of their learning, they take responsibility for what they learn, and they are not particularly inclined to learn something in which they have no interest, or in which they do not see a meaning or purpose.

Adult education is not simply about processing information, as cognitivism suggested, nor is it about observing changes in individual behavior in the face of changes in the environment, as behaviorism indicated, according to the logic of response to a stimulus.

Among the various currents that have given their vision and definition of learning, Kolb's [23] theory of experiential learning, which we will examine in more detail in the next paragraph, takes on particular importance for the adult learner in a Simulation Centre.

The courses of a Simulation Centre generally involve health professionals who have a working approach matured over the years, which derives from their specific life and professional experience, from their university training, often with subsequent specialization in an area of medicine or nursing sciences, and who have been carrying out their profession for many years with excellent results and satisfaction. So what they are approaching to learn is nothing new.

The aim of simulation, which is rooted in the theoretical premise of Knowles' [20] andragogy, is to offer a verisimilar experience that allows one to move from performing automatisms, "because in my department it is always done this way," to being aware of them and being willing to leave some behind. It is necessary to abandon certain comforts in order to go further. For the purposes of this awareness, it is useful for the learner to receive feedback on their performance from peers and the instructor and to actively participate in post-simulation debriefing sessions that are an opportunity to reflect during the process.

Another interesting aspect of learning in a Simulation Centre is that this does not only take place at the level of the individual health worker but also at the level of the group, since it re-proposes what happens in reality: team work, that is, interfacing with colleagues, with operators of other professions and learning to interact by making a "team" function at its best, always with a view to reducing errors and promoting the health and safety of the patient.

The learning process takes place when the learner is willing to question his/her acquired competences and of which he/she is aware, to start a process of re-discussion, experiencing those competences of which he/she is unaware and acquiring not only notions, but more awareness.

1.2.1 Experiential Learning: The Kolb Cycle

Confucius said that "there are three ways to learn wisdom: the first by reflection, the noblest method; the second by imitation, the easiest method; and the third by experience, the bitterest method."

Experience can sometimes be bitter, especially if it is associated with unpleasant feelings, or linked to defeats or mistakes. This is why the noble art of reflection is needed to rehabilitate it. In fact, if we talk about experience, as the central theme for adult learning, we must first dispel a myth: not all experience is transformed into learning. There are so many situations where it is not enough to have lived through them, even if repeatedly, to say that we have learnt. We need a critical analysis to promote learning and personal development following an experience.

According to the most recent neurobiological studies, our brain acquires concepts, notions, and relationships much faster if it is pushed to put them into practice, if it lives them in first person; in fact, the physical and emotional involvement facilitates attention and memory. Our cognition is strictly based on experience and encompasses all the information coming from sensory, imaginative, linguistic, affective, and motivational systems, in order to build a reliable knowledge of an event or a process.

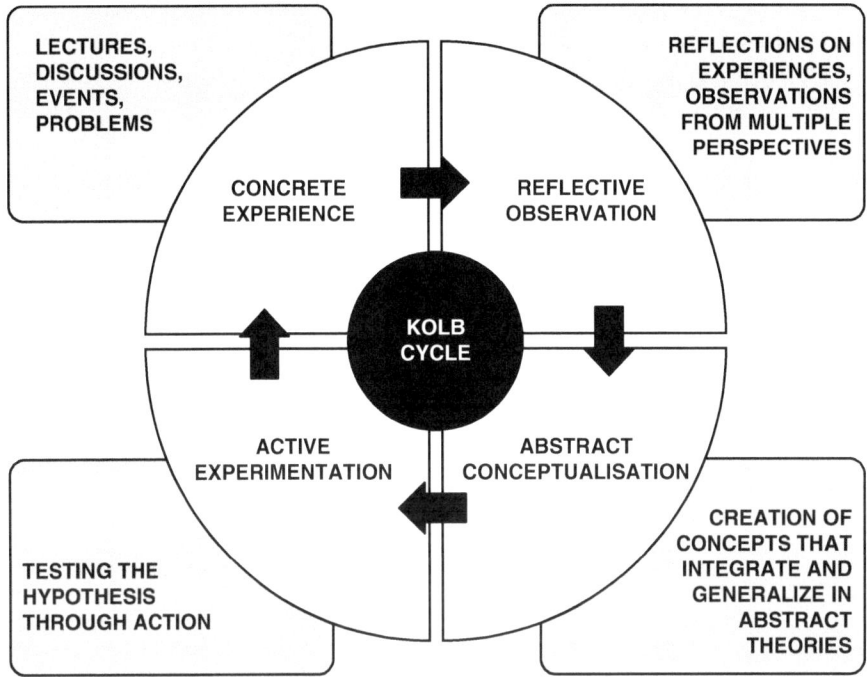

Fig. 1.3 The Kolb cycle

These are the foundations on which experiential learning has developed.

Talent alone is not enough, just as experience alone is not enough: accumulating it does not lead to greater learning, but it is the critical analysis we make of it that leads us toward change.

Experience and reflection are part of a cyclical journey that is described by Kolb's [23] theory of *experiential learning* (Fig. 1.3), a famous American educator who describes experiential learning as an opportunity for learners to acquire and apply knowledge, skills, and attitudes in an immediate and relevant context.

Experiential learning suggests that concrete experience, reflective observation, and active participation are essential elements for the learner to assimilate new knowledge and skills in order to then act appropriately and safely in real clinical situations [24]. Learning is a process in which knowledge is created through observation and transformation of experience, following critical reflection on actions.

Simulation in health education is clearly an example of experiential learning as we can test our learning by repeating simulation scenarios multiple times and reviewing critical situations when debriefing.

The Kolb cycle, applied to training based on simulation, begins with the concrete experience that is a simulated scenario, in which the trainees who participate are involved in the direct execution of a team task that involves the solution of a problem. In the next phase, which is that of observation and reflection, the protagonists of the scenario take part in the debriefing: the concrete experience just performed is reflected upon and analyzed through the narration of the participants' experiences, with questions and observations from the debriefer and any observers.

The debriefing is the moment of "reflective observation" after the experience, where we are asked to give a transformative meaning to our reflections and where the participant takes note of his own limits and resources and becomes more aware of his own attitudes.

Starting from these new understandings, participants are asked to identify the mental schemes and basic assumptions that guided them in the scenario, facilitating the third phase of forming abstract concepts, which integrate experience with theories.

Thanks to the new abstract concepts that the learner will have built up, we arrive at the fourth phase, that of active experimentation, where the learners are asked to experiment the new attitudes on the next occasions in order to transfer the lessons learned to their own working reality and context. This reflection on the action and process experienced during the simulation should lead to a prefiguration of future scenarios and the application of what has been learned.

Each problematic situation addressed during a simulation shows the learner's perception of a difficulty, its identification and definition, the hypothesis of a possible solution, the consideration of the possible consequences of that hypothesis, and the subsequent observations or tests that lead to the acceptance or rejection of the hypothesis [21].

If the experience of the learner is the focus of this learning model, we must also stress the importance and richness of the experience of a good facilitator who can add value to the simulation.

1.2.2   Learning from the Experience of the Other: Mirror Neurons

After seeing the importance of experience and reflection for adult education, we propose a reflection on the process of imitation since the adult also learns from the experience of others.

Through imitation, in fact, individuals are able to convert an observed behavior into a kind of acted behavior, with the ability to put it into action.

According to the theory of mirror neurons, postulated in the late 1990s, thanks to the discovery of Rizzolati and his team of researchers in Neuroscience at the University of Parma, our brain at the sight of an action performed by another person replicates, within itself, that same action, giving rise to what has been called "embodied simulation" [25].

Researchers conducted an experiment on macaques: they had activated electrodes inserted into the neurons of the cerebral cortex with the aim of studying the neural activity of the animal while it was grasping objects. The discovery came when a researcher, entering the animal's room, took a grape, and at the same time, the neurons of the premotor cortex of the monkey, which was watching him, were activated as if the animal itself had grabbed the grapes. In other words, the same part of the brain that is activated in planning a movement is also activated in seeing another individual perform the same series of actions.

This observation led to the discovery of a new type of motor neurons that have the characteristic of responding even in the absence of movement, just by observing an action performed by another subject, hence the name "mirror neurons," since they have the characteristic of encoding not a movement but an intention [26].

Subsequent research has demonstrated the existence of this type of neuron also in humans.

In the light of this theory, one can consider adult learning in a Simulation Centre as learning also acquired by observation and imitation, and it opens a debated topic among the various Simulation Centers: the role of observers. If scenarios are set up for small group work, can they be observed by simple observers, and can they also learn by observing and reflecting on the work of others?

The answer we have given ourselves is that learners learn not only when they simulate but also when they observe, if their observation is finalized and guided by the instructor. However, it is necessary that the observation of others' actions and feelings be followed by participation in the analysis and critical reflection phase, i.e., that observers also participate in the debriefing.

The theory of mirror neurons, according to which they respond equally when an action is performed and when it is observed, could partly explain the role of learning by observation alone, an interesting challenge to previous theories of experiential learning in simulation. According to this theory, the learner learns not only when they themselves simulate but also when they observe others simulate and participate as an active observer in post-simulation debriefing, as Weinstock argues "simulation is nothing more than an excuse to debrief well" [27].

When we see others take part in a simulation scenario, we are also activated from an operational, reflective, and emotional point of view; we share with each other actions, emotions, and feelings, and if we have observed a learner who has felt in great difficulty during a simulation, we too will perceive some degree of difficulty in feeling that emotion.

A simulation thus implies not only a mental representation of what is happening but also an empathic involvement: the emotional states of others imply a projection of self onto the other and a simulation and imitation of action and feeling.

Putting oneself in the other's shoes, feeling what the other is feeling, belongs to the concept of empathy which could be translated in terms of "internal simulation" of the other's emotional states.

Understanding the emotions, intentions, and moods of others and the ability to empathize with peers are extremely important in educational simulation.

Being involved in the processes of understanding the behavior and intentions of others and in the identification of the "what" and "why" of an action, mirror neurons are therefore a master pathway for the processing of simulations at the basis of social cognition [28].

1.2.3   Protected Learning and Psychological Safety

I learned that people can forget what you said, people can forget what you did, but people will never forget how you made them feel. (Maya Angelou)

When an adult chooses for various reasons to participate in medical simulations, knowing the rules of engagement, he does so knowing that this can offer him a number of advantages. In particular, he knows that he can learn something more or less complex without putting himself or even a real patient at risk.

However, simulating implies a risk that the adult may have difficulty managing: acting "as if" means in fact questioning oneself in front of others, whether they are one's peers, other offspring, or the facilitator. This difficulty of the learner has various implications and should not be underestimated but respected, valued, and above all protected.

An adult has now built his own image and identity through complex balances that he needs to continually reconfirm. The image that comes from interaction with others is a fundamental source of reassurance, but it can also be a source of non-confirmation and is therefore usually protected with roles and behaviors that act as screens.

While we simulate, many of these screens are temporarily suspended to put on the role of the learner, and this exposes the adult and makes him more vulnerable than in normal, real life. The management of the "return of image" that the adult has during the learning through simulation is very complex and delicate.

It is necessary to provide the adult learner with a protected learning environment that gives him/her the best chance of learning. The need to have a positive self-image, to appreciate oneself, and to be appreciated by others is a primary need of the adult learner.

The maintenance of a positive self-image is unfortunately not always guaranteed by the traditional educational method, which is based on the learner's acknowledgement of the error made and on which a whole series of feedbacks revolves in which the attention of both the learner and the teacher is monopolized by the negative aspects of the presentation.

This is why we talk about "protected learning" or "safe learning" because a Simulation Centre must ensure that training takes place in a safe environment both physically and psychologically.

In simulation, a protected environment is created when you have succeeded in making participants understand that whatever you do, it will still have some value to you and others.

Psychological safety does not necessarily equate to comfort, but rather to the fact that participants feel free to express even their own moments of discomfort, with the security of being listened to, welcomed, without the feeling of being judged, humiliated, or belittled by either the other learners or the facilitator.

In fact, the facilitator must be able to convey both explicitly (verbal communication) and implicitly (nonverbal communication, attitudes) a sense of psychological safety, i.e., the feeling that the mistakes made during a simulation are an opportunity to learn and a resource for learning and not a cause of embarrassment or punitive consequences.

This basic assumption should be remembered and agreed upon in the "psychological safety pact" between learners and facilitators, along with the notion of confidentiality, explicitly reminding participants that their individual performances and reflections in the debriefings are not intended to be shared outside the Simulation Centre. Indeed, confidentiality is absolutely necessary to facilitate the immediate establishment of the relationship of trust and transparency between facilitators and learners that can help promote fearless participation by learners.

The experience of simulation can be new for some people and already in itself arouse a certain degree of tension. It is certainly full of emotions, which may be both pleasant and less pleasant such as those of performance anxiety, feeling judged, or under stress (even if we are simulating, the emotions are real).

The psychological well-being of the learners must be ensured as having a good state of mind is essential to being prepared for learning.

Questioning oneself can happen in a debriefing situation, and that is why participants are always solicited and stimulated to express doubts and feelings to better manage them without denying them. We can, therefore, neither foresee nor avoid the fact that there are learners who feel certain feelings, and we can only invite them to communicate them to the group or to the facilitator.

1.3   Training Methods: From Frontal Lesson to Simulation

Developing an educational program is complex. There are various factors to take into account as the training methods for simulation vary according to the educational objectives.

The training methods adopted in a Simulation Centre are generally developed following a series of learning stages. Before the course, the learner can receive handouts on which to study and review the topics of the simulations. This allows in advance for the familiarization with theories or algorithms of reference that could be recalled during the simulations.

In the early stages of a simulation-based course, learners acquire factual knowledge about the content of an activity: they are told what they need to know in order to be able to perform a particular action. With practice and familiarization with the Centre, factual knowledge is gradually transformed into automatic behaviors and skills that require less attention and awareness.

Case studies and *role-playing* are suitable tools in the early stages of training where the learners begin to put themselves in the shoes of the role required and gradually expose themselves to the training. Reflecting on the work of others has the advantage of not directly exposing the learner to judgement, as it is the first time he or she has had the time to identify and understand how it works. The general objective, however, should not be to learn to simulate in order to simulate, but to learn to transfer the knowledge and awareness learned by simulating into one's own work context.

Before embarking on team simulation, it is advisable and recommended that the learner not only possesses the content and skills but has learned to work in a team. The premise for a teamwork is in fact "building the group," moving from having a group of experts to an expert group, because the sum is very often, as Gestalt suggests, something more than the simple sum of the parts.

For this reason, many activities are propaedeutic for simulation, and it would be very appropriate to start simulating only after having mastered and acquired, in a stable way, both the single technical skills and the dynamics of group functioning. It is possible to make small experiments of group dynamics, communication, and using *serious games* suitable to the objectives of the specific learning.

While a defibrillator may have the same type of operation and instructions regardless of which department it is placed in, the unit is a "working device" that you may know in theory but in practice then takes on different connotations and facets.

Once learners have acquired the basic knowledge and are familiar with the aptitudes needed for a given activity, it is essential that they practice their skills.

In classroom training, the choice of teaching methodology must take into account the need to arouse the interest of the participants and the recovery and sharing of their experiences, so mistakes as well as experiences can be put to capital.

The frontal lesson can be useful to break the ice, to transmit some basic concepts, and is always useful to recall the theory: it is, however, functional to the learning and to the maintenance of the level of attention to alternate moments of theory with moments of practice. It is important to avoid the debriefing becoming a review of theoretical concepts; if this need emerges during the debriefing, take some time later to review some topics.

The team simulation is approached gradually, considering both individual exercises and exercises in pairs and small groups, in a crescendo of complexity and cooperation.

Teaching and training are not the antithesis of learning; they are a complement to it, and they are configured less and less as an indoctrination of contents and more and more as a support for learning a method of reading and analyzing facts.

Simulation is the ideal training method for the experiential learning we described above, as it provides opportunities for interprofessional collaboration, facilitating the comparison of the specific knowledge of each professional category, thus leading to the improvement of the understanding of different roles and the achievement of *problem-solving* skills [29].

Simulation will never be able to fully replace patient-facing care experiences in a real-world clinical setting, but it still manages to provide a care approach that is superimposed on the real thing, with the advantage of being carried out in a controlled environment allowing learners to make mistakes, without them resulting in consequences [29, 30].

1.4   Elements and Characteristics of Communication

Communication is the foundation of all human relationships, and although we use it every day, we are not always aware of the logic behind it, the processes it triggers, and the incredible potential it has.

The term communication derives from the Latin *com*, i.e., "with," and "munire," i.e., "to bind," *and* in its original meaning, it means "to share," i.e., to share thoughts, opinions, experiences, sensations, and feelings with others. Communication, which therefore involves two or more individuals, indicates a series of phenomena involving the transfer of information and is based on a relationship in which the interlocutors influence each other, even if they are not aware of it.

The debriefer must be a good communicator: he/she must involve the trainees, stimulate them, make them participate, and motivate them; and he/she must be able to transmit, in an effective and clear way, the contents of the training session. However, the debriefer must also understand that it is impossible not to communicate. According to Watzlawick et al. [31], any behavior communicates something. No matter how hard we try to be silent and passive, we are still sending a message, i.e., the will not to communicate with others. Communication can in fact be involuntary, unintentional, and unconscious. As a facilitator, therefore, with the responsibility of conducting a reflective conversation after the scenario, which is the adult's real learning moment, it is important to know the elements and techniques of communication and at the same time be aware of the need to constantly adjust communication according to the objectives, the context, and the type of relationship with different individuals.

Communication is a process during which several subjects interact and carry out actions aimed at producing, transmitting, interpreting, and understanding messages with a specific purpose and based on shared rules. The elements of communication are those parts that constitute communicative sequences and allow the transmission of content. These elements are multiple and should be considered as interrelated. According to the linear model of explanation of the communicative process of Shannon and Weaver [32], in a communicative sequence, we distinguish (a) the sender, i.e., respectively, the person who communicates the message; (b) the receiver, i.e., the single person or several recipients of the message itself; (c) the message, i.e., the content of what is communicated which may be information, data, news, or more simply a feeling; (d) the code, i.e., the system of signs that is used when communicating and without which the message cannot be transmitted and may be represented by a language, a gesture, a graph, or a drawing; and (e) the channel, understood both as the technical means external to the subject by which the message arrives (telephone, fax, mail, etc.) and as the sensory means involved in the transmission of the message. Sender and receiver perform two important actions:

the first encodes, i.e., transforms ideas, concepts, and mental images into a communicable message through the code, and in parallel, the second performs decoding, i.e., transforms the message from code into ideas, concepts, and mental images. Finally, there is the (f) context or environment, that is, the place, physical or social, where the communicative exchange takes place [32]. In every type of communication, there is also a form of noise (g), i.e., the irrelevant information that makes the passage of the signal difficult (e.g., background noise in an environment). Noise produces loss of information. Each element affects the success of the communication, and the probability that everything will work properly is very low in most human communications.

It is also important to know and learn how to effectively use all levels of communication. Specifically, three levels are recognized:

- Verbal, which indicates the content of what is said and concerns the choice of words and the logical construction of sentences, according to grammatical and syntactic structures.
- Nonverbal, which concerns everything that is conveyed through movements and posture, the position one occupies in space, and aesthetic aspects. It therefore includes gestures, looks, facial expressions, hand position, and clothing.
- Paraverbal, which refers to the way something is expressed, i.e., the tone, volume, and rhythm of the voice but also pauses, silence, and other sound expressions, such as laughter or simply clearing one's throat.

We cannot, therefore, send a message of content without at the same time co-sending an affective-emotional message of relationship. In some cases, it is even estimated that nonverbal and paraverbal communication is decisive in at least 93% of the message transmitted [33]. It is therefore important for the debriefer to also know how to listen actively to their students, paying attention to their verbal-textual modes of expression.

As Galileo Galilei had already warned us when he said that "good teaching is one quarter preparation and three quarters theatre," communication is therefore not only what we say but also how we say it, when we say it, and includes what we do not say.

Since the debriefer's work is based on interpersonal relationships and communication, it is important, for the training experience to be effective, to know the three styles of communication:

- Assertive: he or she actively listens by asking questions to check that he or she has understood; expresses his or her own thoughts and emotions while always respecting the individuality and point of view of others; asks politely and firmly to continue if interrupted; is available for dialogue and comparison and to reach an agreement with the other interlocutors; and affirms himself or herself without devaluing or overestimating others.

- Aggressive: this is assumed by those who use an arrogant tone of voice, show no interest in others, are bad listeners, do not respect the ideas of other interlocutors, impose their own convictions without the possibility of negotiation, and constantly interrupt, even going so far as to verbally attack.
- Passive: characterized by hesitation in expressing one's own ideas, in being afraid of being heard and judged, in using a submissive and insecure voice, and in the belief that other interlocutors are always better.

References

1. Reason, J. (2000). Human error: Models and management. *British Medical Journal, 320,* 768–770.
2. Rasmussen, J. (1986). *Information processing and human-machine interaction: An approach to cognitive engineering.* North-Holland.
3. Reason, J. (1994). *Human error.* il Mulino.
4. Reason, J. (1990). *Human error.* Cambridge University Press.
5. Wheelan, S. A., Burchill, C. N., & Tilin, F. (2003). The link between teamwork and patients' outcomes in intensive care units. *American Journal of Critical Care, 12*(6), 527–534.
6. Reason, J. T. (2008). *The human contribution: Unsafe acts, accidents and heroic recoveries.* Ashgate Publishing.
7. Weick, K. E. (1991). The non-traditional quality of organizational learning. *Organization Science, 2*(1), 116–124.
8. Chialastri, A. (2011). *Human factor.* IBN.
9. Kohn, L. T., Corrigan, J. M., Donaldson, J. M., & Institute of Medicine (US) Committee on Quality of Health Care in America. (2000). *To err is human building a safer health system.* National Academies Press.
10. Flin, R., Youngson, G., & Yule, S. (2007). How do surgeons make intraoperative decisions? *BMJ Quality and Safety, 16*(3), 235–239.
11. Koonce, J. M. (2002). *Human factors in the training of pilots.* CRC Press.
12. Wiener, E. L. (1993). *Intervention strategies for the management of human error.* ntrs. nasa.gov
13. Gaba, D. M., Fish, K. J., & Howard, S. K. (1994). *Crisis management in anesthesiology.* Churchill Livingstone.
14. DeKeyser, V., & Woods, D. D. (1990). Fixation errors: Failures to revise situation assessment in dynamic and risky systems. In A. G. Colombo & A. S. Bustamante (Eds.), *Systems reliability assessment.* Kluwer.
15. Grillo, V. (2015, October 23–25). *From error prevention to safety promotion. An ongoing experience.* XIII Congresso Nazionale Sis 118, Cosenza.
16. Corrado, F. (2019). *In praise of failure.* Sperling & Kupfer.
17. Kothari, L. G., Shah, K., & Barach, P. (2017). Simulation based medical education in graduate medical education training and assessment programs. *Progress in Pediatric Cardiology, 44,* 33–42.
18. Maran, N. J., & Glavin, R. J. (2003). Low-to high-fidelity simulation-a continuum of medical education? *Medical Education, 37,* 22–28.
19. Wang, E. E. (2011). Simulation and adult learning. *Disease-a-Month, 57*(11), 664–678.
20. Knowles, M. (1993). *When the adult learns. Pedagogy and andragogy* (Vol. 6). Franco Angeli.
21. Dewey, J., Borghi, L., & Ratner, J. (1961). *Today's education.* New Italy.
22. Rogers, C. R., & Freiberg, H. J. (1969). *Freedom to learn.* Charles E. Merrill.
23. Kolb, D. A. (1984). *Experiential learning: Experience as the source of learning and development.* Prentice-Hall.

24. Zannini, L. (2005). *Tutorship in adult education: A pedagogical look* (Vol. 32). Guerini Scientific.
25. Ferrari, P. F., & Gallese, V. (2007). Mirror neurons and intersubjectivity. *Advances in Consciousness Research, 68*, 73.
26. Rizzolatti, G., & Sinigaglia, C. (2006). *I know what you do: The acting brain and mirror neurons*. Raffaello Cortina Publisher.
27. Weinstock, P. (2013). *Boston children's hospital simulator program, simulation instructor workshop. Personal communication*. Harvard University.
28. Anolli, L., & Mantovani, F. (2011). *How our mind works. Learning, simulation and serious games*. il Mulino.
29. Titzer, J. L., Swenty, C. F., & Hoehn, W. G. (2012). An interprofessional simulation promoting collaboration and problem solving among nursing and allied health professional students. *Clinical Simulation in Nursing, 8*(8), e325–e333.
30. Sponton, A., & Iadeluca, A. (2014). *Simulation in nursing: Methodologies, techniques and strategies for teaching*. Ambrosiana Publishing House.
31. Watzlawick, P., Beavin, J. H., & Jackson, D. D. (1971). *Pragmatics of human communication*. Astrolabe.
32. Shannon, C. E., & Weaver, W. (1949). *A mathematical theory of communication*. University of Illinois Press.
33. Mehrabian, A. (1981). *Silent messages: Implicit communication of emotions and attitudes*. Wadsworth.

> *Intelligence is not to make no mistakes, but quickly to see*
> *how to make them good.*
>
> Bertolt Brecht

2.1 Definition of Debriefing

Debriefing is the analytical process used to reflect on the actions performed during the scenario. It is grounded in Kolb's theory of experiential learning, according to which learning among adults is based on the conscious reflection of experience and not on experience per se [1].

There are numerous definitions of debriefing attributable to various authors who have studied the topic. "Debriefing provides an opportunity to explore and make sense of what happened during an event or experience, discussing what went well and identifying what could be done to change, improve, and do better next time" [2].

It involves "the active participation of learners, guided by a facilitator or instructor whose primary goal is to identify and fill gaps in knowledge and skills" [3]. Debriefing has also been referred to as a facilitated post-event analysis meeting, also generally defined as a "non-judgmental, participant-centered technique to help a professional or team improve their performance through reflective practice" [4].

If simulation is a particular learning method, debriefing is its essential pivot, to such an extent that all agree that debriefing in simulation is such an essential part of the learning process that it should never be omitted [5] and that a simulation without debriefing should not exist, as "the simulation itself is the excuse to debrief" [2, 6]. For others, even simulation without adequate debriefing would be "ineffective and even unethical" [7]. According to Dieckmann et al. [8], "post-scenario debriefing is important to maximize learning and facilitate change at the individual and systemic level, modifying for the better one's attitudes, perceptions, behaviors, actions and technical skills, organization culture, policies, procedures, and operational mechanisms." Without this post-event guided process, reflection on what participants learned would be largely left to chance, making the simulation less effective [9].

As we will see in Sect. 2.7, debriefing is not synonymous with feedback. In contrast to simple feedback, debriefing is something different and sometimes more complex. In fact, feedback is a unidirectional transmission of information to the

G. Capogna et al., *Strategic Debriefing for Advanced Simulation*,
https://doi.org/10.1007/978-3-031-06104-2_2

learner about his/her performance during the simulation. Debriefing, on the other hand, is an interactive, bidirectional, reflective discussion, or conversation about the practiced practice.

Debriefing thus becomes a constitutive and supporting element of the medical simulation educational model and is recommended by guidelines [10], and its effectiveness is confirmed by numerous studies and systematic reviews [11–17].

2.2   Purpose of Debriefing and Learning Objectives

The purpose of the debriefing is to engage participants in a reflective discussion about their performance in relation to the learning objectives on which the simulation experience was designed, enriched by other important points or events that may have occurred.

There is no debriefing or any other form of feedback without learning objectives, i.e., those cognitive (the knowledge) and operational and social skills (the know-how) that the participants will acquire or on which they will be able to reflect through participation in the case.

Even a simple task like stacking bricks is supported by learning objectives, and learners should receive at least some feedback regarding the technique they used and the time it took to complete the exercise. The objectives, thus, will inform the primary debriefing discussion and the take-home learning messages. At the end of a simulation, the debriefer should already have a plan in mind with the topics to be discussed because, when the scenario is ended, he or she usually has just a few minutes to gather ideas and begin debriefing. The discussion can be directed either at the learning objectives of the scenario established earlier or at the participants' newly observed performance. Very often, in fact, due to the unforeseen behavior of the participants themselves or simply by chance, it can happen that new learning points emerge, which obviously require the debriefer's maximum attention, since, as already stated, the educational process starts from the needs of the learners and not from those of the debriefer. Any events or deficiencies in performance related to patient safety should always and in any case be explored in accordance with the concept of "learner-centered debriefing" [18], whereby debriefing points pre-identified during the scenario design phase need not be rigidly adhered to, and other points may instead be discussed if judged more important to all the learners participating in the simulation session.

When the simulation aims to promote team training involving a multi-professional team, it is important to discuss objectives that may engage the majority of the team, such as strategies that could have been adopted to effectively improve communication during the scenario. Otherwise, the risk would be to focus exclusively on technical skills objectives that involve only a particular discipline or even a specific health professional. In some cases, debriefing goals can be identified during the debriefing itself, e.g., during the "reaction phase" when emotions are shared (the feeling of confusion reported by all participants upon exiting the scenario most likely underlies a general communication deficit in the team to be explored during debriefing) or during the "descriptive phase" (the discrepancy in understanding of the case diagnosis between the *leader* and the team hides ineffective communication). This possibility to collect the debriefing objectives "in progress," that is, "also during" the debriefing itself, forces the debriefer to listen carefully to what is said with an open mind, paying particular attention to what participants have to say, ready to catch any criticality that could turn out to be a resource for the discussion. "Most people listen with the intention of answering, not with the desire to understand" (AC Doyle): one of the traps into which the novice debriefer falls is to prepare the next question while the learner is answering his previous question. In this way, he fails to listen and take the opportunity to elaborate with another relevant question.

Often, there are so many topics to be discussed during the debriefing that there is a risk of quickly exceeding the allotted time and the learners' ability to reflect. It is therefore more convenient to prioritize and choose no more than two, three, or four main points to cover. Otherwise, the benefit of debriefing may be compromised, as participants may be so overloaded that they may not retain, except superficially, what they have learned. Although it is theoretically reported that five to nine topics may be the ideal number in order not to exceed the threshold of working memory capacity [19], in practice, a good debriefer will be satisfied when each of the participants has understood and internalized at least one learning point such that it can be the building block of a change for the better in his/her clinical practice.

2.3   Debriefing Participants

The participants in a debriefing are usually the debriefer (possibly accompanied by a co-debriefer) and those who participated in the scenario (learners, actors, and staff who took part in the simulation).

Sometimes, when you have to facilitate a debriefing that contains many technical issues that the debriefer is not competent in, you can use an expert in the field who can attend the scenario from the control room or from a nearby room with a live streaming audio and video and who can intervene in the debriefing conversation to clarify the more properly technical aspects when requested by the debriefer.

In principle, the scenario and the debriefing should always be considered as a personal and confidential educational experience and therefore subject to the rules of privacy and respect for confidentiality. However, in some cases, the scenario can be observed by "passive" participants (who do not practice the scenario), usually from a nearby room with live audio and video streaming, and they can be subsequently involved in the debriefing process. In this case, it is even more important that the debriefer extends the basic rules of debriefing to the observers, for example, be respectful, do not judge, raise your hand for questions, etc. The presence of outside observers should always be communicated to the scenario participants so that they can give their explicit consent to be observed by third parties not directly involved in the scenario.

2.4   When, Where, and How Long to Debrief

Theoretically, from a time perspective, debriefing can occur either after the completion of the scenario ("post-event debriefing") or during the scenario ("in-event debriefing"), but the best and most commonly used time is the facilitator-led post-scenario debriefing [2] (Fig. 2.1).

It is important that the facilitator who will conduct the debriefing asks participants to remain silent from the end of the scenario until they are all comfortably seated and ready to debrief, in order to avoid them sharing their first impressions and reactions only in private. In fact, these initial exchanges are very important and very often relate to emotions, and may not come out easily during the structured reaction phase if they have already been disclosed in private. Coming out from the assigned role is facilitated, in a nonverbal manner, by inviting participants to change and remove the scrubs or uniforms worn during the simulation before the debriefing begins.

It is best for the debriefing to take place in a different room from where the scenario took place, in a comfortable environment, to encourage stepping out of the assigned role and reflection for a number of reasons: (a) the participants continue to look at the "patient" (the mannequin) and equipment and, therefore, may not focus

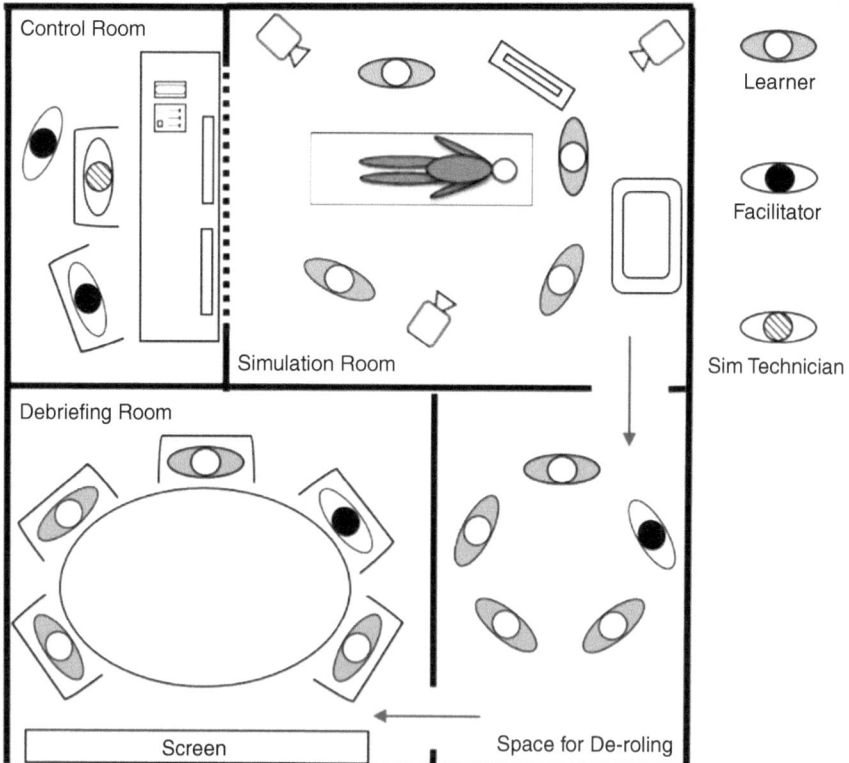

Fig. 2.1 Typical layout of a simulation session

fully on the debriefing; (b) staying in the simulation room could delay the room refitting phase, necessary to start the next scenario; (c) anyone tidying up the environment while the debriefing is still in progress would distract the participants; and (d) changing environment also facilitates the participants to come out of their role in the scenario.

It should also be remembered that the environment in which the debriefing takes place has an overall impact on cognitive load and can be a conditioning factor on learning and performance [20]. It is recommended that the chosen room is free from distracting elements (posters, large windows, background noise, etc.).

Regarding the arrangement of participants in the room where the debriefing takes place, everyone should be seated, comfortably, in a circle [21] to reiterate the fact that the debriefing is fundamentally a circular learning process among adults, non-judgmental and peer to peer. A "classroom"-type arrangement implies, in fact, that the debriefer is in a position of authority or superiority, not in line with the learner-centered educational approach.

The duration of the debriefing depends on the approach adopted, which in turn could be related to the type of simulation and participants involved. Depending on the complexity of the scenario and the number of professionals involved, a debriefing generally lasts 20–45 min [22], which is often equivalent to about twice the duration of the scenario [15].

2.5   Qualities of the Debriefer

The facilitator's role is to serve as a guide to the conversation and to ensure that relevant issues (e.g., learning goals) are discussed and that the conversation flows smoothly and does not go off topic. As described by Fanning and Gaba [23], unlike a traditional "teacher," the facilitator does not pose as an authority or expert, but rather as a *co-learner*.

A debriefer should be trained to facilitate the process of critical reflection using educational, clinical, and technical skills, as well as the human qualities and abilities of a good communicator. Debriefing can, in fact, be counterproductive if the communication technique used is too harsh, rude, or perceived as offensive or authoritarian by participants. The trap is that participants may be forced to take a defensive stance because of the debriefer's wrong attitudes. Unlike the traditional classroom teaching context, the debriefer should position himself or herself as a co-learner, i.e., "sitting among them" rather than in front of them, higher, or standing, and facilitate the debriefing in an exploratory way instead of lecturing. The debriefer as facilitator uses open-ended questions, positive reinforcement, cognitive aids, and audiovisual media to help others analyze, synthesize, evaluate problems, and extrapolate and apply lessons learned to future situations [24]. The debriefer should always consider the participants as intelligent, competent, willing to do their best, eager to improve, and open to learning [25]. He or she should possess educational, clinical, and technical skills, but also some human qualities and skills as good communicators.

2.6   Structure of the Debriefing

Although not standardized, debriefing is commonly divided into a series of phases to ensure that the conversation proceeds in a structured and orderly manner from start to finish.

In general, simulation and post-simulation debriefing are anticipated by the so-called briefing, that is, the period of time when information about an event or task and the context in which it takes place is conveyed to learners in order to facilitate a better understanding of what is expected during the simulation-based experience, including expectations, confidentiality, and times and logistics for the experience [26]. It sets the stage and therefore needs to be well planned. It ensures, in fact, that learners are prepared for the educational content and are aware of the ground rules for following the training experience. It might include initial patient clinical presentation, the past medical history, the participant's role, and all the relevant elements essential to set the stage. During the briefing, the "fiction contract" is established, i.e., the pact between learners and teachers: "you don't pretend, we don't do tricks." In other words, learners are asked to "suspend disbelief" about the potential limitations of simulation [27] and to act as if they were in a real situation, treating the simulator or "patient" with dignity, respect, and professionalism. The briefing also plays a key role in establishing a psychologically safe environment, ensuring that the learners feel comfortable about expressing thoughts without feeling uncomfortable or fearing negative consequences [28].

Many debriefing techniques run through three main phases or more and contain common elements, such as the initial attention to reactions and emotions, descriptions of events, analysis and understanding of performance, synthesis, and take-home message(s).

Dealing with initial reactions and emotions, known as the "reaction" or "stepping out of the role" phase, is intended to give participants time to address reactions and emotions in order to "clear the air" and allow the discussion to proceed with a lighter emotional load. The descriptive phase allows for a description of the events that unfolded, providing a summary of simulation events and the establishment of a shared mental model. This phase, sometimes, includes the clarification of the purpose of the simulation and its learning objectives [29].

The understanding, examining, or analysis phase is devoted to learner-centered reflection: the focus is on what happened during the simulation and why the participants behaved the way they did. During this phase, targeted questions are used to stimulate reflection and expose the learners' thinking.

The synthesis phase focuses on reflecting on what was learned, codifying the insights gained during the analysis phase. During this phase, the debriefer ensures that all important learning objectives have been touched upon and provides a review of lessons learned. In addition, the debriefer encourages learners to describe how they will apply the lessons learned during the debriefing in their future clinical practice.

The different debriefing techniques, their structure, and their characteristics are described in Table 2.1.

Table 2.1 Different debriefing techniques, structure, and characteristics

	Technique	Phases	Description
THREE-PHASE STRUCTURE	RAS (Rudolph et al. 2006)	Reaction Analysis Synthesis	The first phase focuses on exploring reactions and the emotional impact the scenario had on the participants. In this phase, learners can "vent" before completing the rest of the debriefing. During the second phase, the focus is on what happened during the simulation and why the participants behaved the way they did. The third phase focuses on reflecting on what was learned and codifying the insights gained during the analysis phase.
	3D model (Zigmont et al. 2011)	Defusing Discovering Deepening	It consists of three phases. Essentially the function of each of the phases is similar to that described by Rudolph.
	GAS (Phrampus and O'Donnell 2013)	Gather Analyze Synthesis	It consists of three-phases. The first phase encourages the team to provide a summary of simulation events to establish a shared mental model. The second phase is devoted to learner-centered reflection and the analysis of actions during the simulation. During this phase, targeted questions are used to stimulate reflection and expose the learners' thinking. The final phase ensures that all important learning objectives have been touched upon and provides a review of lessons learned
	Diamond method (Jaye et al. 2015)	Description, Analysis Application	The conversational structure in this model includes three phases. The purpose of the first two phases is similar to that described in the GAS model. The application phase focuses specifically on asking participants how they will apply the lessons learned during the debriefing in their clinical practice. This model does not include an actual reaction phase, although participants are generally asked at the beginning of the debriefing "So, what happened" and during the analysis "How did that make you feel?".
	3-R Model (ICISF 2017)	Review Response Remind	Originating from the International Critical Incident Stress Foundation, the model consists of three stages. In the Review phase, the debriefer invites learners to reflect on how they think they did and whether inappropriate actions were carried out. In the following phase, the debriefer explores the concerns of the team members about their own perceptions and performance. In the last phase, the debriefer encourages the learners to recall what they have done.
MULTIPHASE STRUCTURE	RUST (Karlsen 2013)	Reaction Understanding Summary Take-home message	*Promoting Excellence and Reflective Learning in Simulation* method uses a four-stage structure. The first phase - the debriefer asks about the learners' feelings allowing them to vent and express their initial thoughts. In the second phase, the debriefer invites learners to summarize their perspective of key events or major medical events faced during the scenario, to make sure that all are on the same page. In the third phase the debriefer uses one or more techniques to encourage learner self-assessment and to close performance gaps. In the summary phase, the debriefer encourages the learners to state their main take-home message(s)
	TeamGAINS (Kolbe et al. 2013)	Reaction Discussion of the clinic Transition from simulation to reality Discussion of behavioral skills Synthesis Supervision of practice	*Team-Guided Team Self-Correction, Advocacy-Inquiry, and Systemic-Constructivist* include six sequential phases. The systemic-constructivist techniques used in TeamGAINS focus on the individuals within their system and the dynamics of interaction and relationship, rather than the behavior of the individual.
	AAR (Sawyer and Deering, 2013)	D - defining the rules S - explaining learning objectives B - benchmarking performance R - reviewing expected actions I - identifying what happened E - examining why events went that way F - formalizing learning.	The *After Action Review* is based on the U.S. Army's AAR methodology. Using this conversational structure, debriefing proceeds through 7 stages, which can be recalled by the acronym "DEBRIEF". Dividing the debriefing into multiple phases is intended to ensure a shared mental model and to allow participants to objectively compare their performance against a known standard or specific performance benchmark.
	GREAT (Owen & Follows 2006)	G - Guidelines R - Recommendations E - Events A - Analysis T - Transfer	It is a checklist for debriefing, encouraging facilitators to: refer to the most recent best evidence-based guidelines related to scenario management; use reviews where no guidelines exist; allow time for learners to reflect on the simulation to identify key events; help participants go through a detailed analysis of their performance; and help participants identify what learning they will be able to apply to their clinical practice. GREAT is not presented in chronological order, but instead, the facilitator is often asked to jump back and forth between the different elements while analyzing the different parts of the scenarios.

(continued)

Table 2.1 (continued)

MULTIPHASE STRUCTURE			
	LEARN (Sigalet et al. 2017)	L - Learning objectives E - Emotions A and R - Actions and Reflections N - Next steps	Debriefing for Meaningful Learning model is reminiscent of the Socratic maieutic method and uses six stages for debriefing. The debriefer does not give information but asks the participants a series of questions, and from the answers deep questions are probed.
	DML (Dreifuerst 2015)	Engage Explore Explain Elaborate Evaluate Extend	It is used to help trainers organize an effective educational feedback session: trainers should firstly review the learning objectives in light of the observed performance deficits; then they should ask learners to express emotions associated with the simulation; (A) and (R) Actions and Reflections: for which various approaches can be used, such as directive feedback, delta/plus, etc.; finally, the facilitator asks learners to identify one thing they learned from the session that they will put into practice next time.
	PEARLS (Bajaj et al. 2018)	Reactions Description Analysis Application/summary	It is used to help trainers organize an effective educational feedback session: trainers should firstly review the learning objectives in light of the observed performance deficits; then they should ask learners to express emotions associated with the simulation; (A) and (R) Actions and Reflections: for which various approaches can be used, such as directive feedback, delta/plus, etc.; finally, the facilitator asks learners to identify one thing they have learned from the session that they will put into practice next time.

2.7   Communication Methods Used in Debriefing

There are many possible communicative approach methods that can be used for debriefing discussion [29]. We will examine the most commonly used in healthcare: directive feedback and self-feedback, which are one-way approaches; the plus/delta method, which is a process-centered approach; and facilitation, focused on advocating one's own positions and seeing the views of others (assertion-inquiry), which positions the debriefer as a cognitive detective. To these must be added the strategic, change-focused approach, which will be discussed, in detail, in Chaps. 4 and 5.

2.7.1   Feedback (Directive, Peer, and Self-feedback)

Feedback is a one-way communication approach from the facilitator to learners about their behavior. Feedback and debriefing are often used interchangeably, although they are not synonymous, feedback being a unidirectional process of information transfer [30, 31] and not a two-way, interactive conversation.

Feedback comes in many shapes and forms. The Healthcare Simulation Dictionary defines it as "an activity in which information is relayed back to the learner, based on his or her performance during an observed activity or its outcome" [32]. Thus, it is not an actual debriefing, but rather a communication strategy that can be used in given situations.

Directive feedback is a didactic report provided to the learners, which results from the comparison of desired outcome to actual outcome at the end of the simulation. Thus, the "debriefer" here acts more like an instructor rather than a facilitator, and learners are more passive, acting mainly as recipients of information. This approach can be used when performance deficits have to do with technical skills and/or concrete knowledge rather than behavioral concepts. Obviously, directive feedback has several limitations: (1) it does not explore the learner's motivations for action (the mental framework); (2) it risks slipping into a judgmental approach, especially if the instructor has an authoritative stance; (3) it does not truly engage the learner except as a recipient of information, as the process is guided solely by the instructor; and (4) by shortening the discussion, it does not allow for in-depth debate. Furthermore, it can have a negative emotional impact on learners if not carefully integrated [33]. The psychological safety of learners is indeed a priority aspect when deciding to provide directive feedback. In order to mitigate the judgmental nature of such an approach, many educators use the sandwich feedback method, in which positive points are first discussed, then elements in need of improvement are analyzed, and finally strengths are called out again. Although praise generally helps maintain the learner's self-confidence, it would not seem to really improve their future performance [34]. In practice then, it can be said that feedback is a very different form of performance review as it does not clarify the reasons for the participants' actions or thinking; nevertheless, it can be used partially within and at certain points in a debriefing.

A further variation is peer feedback, in which it is the learners themselves who give each other feedback, but this particular type of feedback should only be used after establishing clear ground rules of mutual respect and should still involve the presence of the instructor, who is always ready to take back control of the session. To perform this type of feedback, learners need a certain level of clinical experience and expertise. The last type of feedback is self-reflection, for which no facilitator is required beyond the initial orientation [35]. It requires maturity and discipline on the part of the learners, is usually based on pre-constructed questionnaires, and is an approach used by some for checking non-technical skills [35].

2.7.2   Plus/Delta

In the "plus/delta" method, "plus" are the actions carried out by the individual and/or the team during the scenario deemed as timely and appropriate, and "delta" are the actions which the group of participants or the individual judges deemed as needing improvement [36].

Debriefing plus/delta is therefore a process-focused, facilitator-led debriefing [37]. Participants are asked "What worked in this scenario? What is the best thing you did?" (plus). When all responses seem to be exhausted, the facilitator asks "What could be improved?" or "What could have been done differently or better?" (delta).

This method has several advantages: (1) it is a quick and easy way to debrief; (2) it is learner-driven as they provide their own self-assessment; and (3) many solutions can be proposed in a very short period of time, leading to several suggestions for improvement, especially if, for example, the facilitator asks everyone to write on a sticky note the "plus" and on another the "delta" and then asks them to paste them on a whiteboard. But it also implies disadvantages: (1) it is easy to get lost in the debriefing process if there is no strict rule of how to go through the plus and minus points chronologically; (2) one may miss the opportunity to discuss the intention of the actions, since the "whys" are not investigated; and (3) technically, it is the facilitator who generally suggests how to improve performance deficits [38], and thus the learner's self-reflection is not promoted. Therefore, there is a risk of not changing participants' attitudes but only proposing superficial changes referring to the scenario performed. For this reason, some suggest using this method at the beginning of the analytical phase to identify critical issues in a non-judgmental way, and then use it as a bridge to different methods that delve more deeply into the causes and mental attitudes of learners (plus/delta/plus method) [39].

The plus/delta method can also be used to engage the observers more, by asking them to take notes during the scenario. This allows for the participation of an active observer audience whose suggestions can be used during the debriefing.

2.7.3 Assertion-Investigation

It is a communication technique for exploring participants' performance gaps through the use of questions to discover the reasons behind the actions, so facilitating a non-judgmental debriefing. This technique, known as "advocacy-inquiry" technique, an English term derived from legal language, indicating the analogy with a good defense lawyer who serves the client's interests by investigating the mental processes that led him or her to act in a certain way.

Based on the observed results, the debriefer helps learners explore and uncover the frames that led them to carry out actions in order to improve their performance in similar situations in the future. Advocacy is implemented by assertion, observation, or statement. Ideal advocacy combines the actions (or inactions) observed by the debriefer ("I noticed…") with good judgment about their clinical consequences ("I think…"). Inquiry is shown by an attitude of genuine curiosity that leads the learners to reflect on and share the frames that underlay their actions ("I wonder…").

The assertion-inquiry conversational technique [40] is widely employed, with many variations, in the so-called debriefing with good judgment introduced in 2006 by the Harvard team [41]: The facilitator acts as an external observer who has to identify actions that deserve intervention but to maximize learning is more interested in the mechanisms that generated them.

2.8   Debriefing and Structural Deficits
            in the Working Environment

A particular type of debriefing aimed at identifying latent structural deficits that may induce or facilitate clinical errors within a hospital environment during its testing or construction has recently been described [42].

This type of debriefing has been called by the acronym SAFEE (*Summarize, Anchor, Facilitate, Explore, and Elicit*). The debriefing is preceded by a

Table 2.2 SAFEE debriefing stages

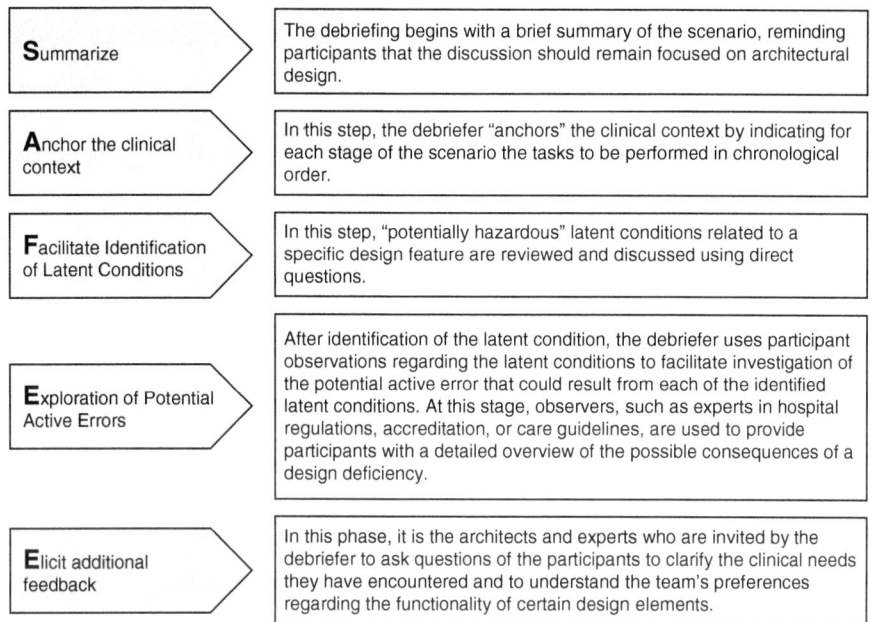

Summarize	The debriefing begins with a brief summary of the scenario, reminding participants that the discussion should remain focused on architectural design.
Anchor the clinical context	In this step, the debriefer "anchors" the clinical context by indicating for each stage of the scenario the tasks to be performed in chronological order.
Facilitate Identification of Latent Conditions	In this step, "potentially hazardous" latent conditions related to a specific design feature are reviewed and discussed using direct questions.
Exploration of Potential Active Errors	After identification of the latent condition, the debriefer uses participant observations regarding the latent conditions to facilitate investigation of the potential active error that could result from each of the identified latent conditions. At this stage, observers, such as experts in hospital regulations, accreditation, or care guidelines, are used to provide participants with a detailed overview of the possible consequences of a design deficiency.
Elicit additional feedback	In this phase, it is the architects and experts who are invited by the debriefer to ask questions of the participants to clarify the clinical needs they have encountered and to understand the team's preferences regarding the functionality of certain design elements.

specially constructed scenario to investigate structural deficits, in which healthcare professionals participate in the role of "frontline participants" and technical staff, such as architects, quality managers, infection control, personnel, etc., in the role of "observers." The debriefing is set up so that design team members understand the operational perspectives of the clinicians in order to identify latent structural errors that may help facilitate active errors in the conduct of a clinical scenario.

The acronym SAFEE summarizes the five phases of this type of debriefing as shown in Table 2.2.

2.9   The Co-debriefing

A "co-debriefing" is defined as when the debriefing is conducted by more than one facilitator. Having one debriefer and one co-debriefer may be helpful in the case of a multi-professional team debriefing, as the two debriefers may have different professional skills and therefore be better able to address the multidisciplinary technical aspects. Debriefing arrangements should be previously agreed upon by the two debriefers at the time of session planning to ensure a unified experience for the learners and consistency (educational approach, debriefing structure, communicative method, scope of topics to be covered for the debriefing—technical vs. non-technical, medical vs. nursing, or any other choice) and to prevent any issues of disagreements during the debriefing itself.

Table 2.3 Benefits and disadvantages of co-debriefing

CO-DEBRIEFING

Benefits	Disadvantages
• Debriefers can be complementary in debriefing style, making for a very engaging discussion • Debriefers can be complementary in expertise and experience • Having two debriefers brings additional perspectives to the case. • A debriefer can prevent the other from forgetting to ask questions of a participant because of the significant cognitive load on him/her for conducting the debriefing • Debriefers can support each other when debriefing is difficult and many performance deficits need to be addressed • The other debriefer may help clarify a point by rephrasing the other debriefer's point • The other debriefer can cross-check participants' understanding of the points addressed, ensuring that performance deficits are adequately addressed • Allowing a second debriefer to contribute to the debriefing helps, in general, teacher growth, as an inexperienced debriefer can gain experience through observation of the more experienced colleague • Debriefers can have different technical skills and this is an advantage in the case of multi-professional teams • One of the debriefers can keep track of the time and learning objectives that have been covered or still need to be addressed	• Debriefing can become a poor learning event if there is not good coordination between debriefers • Debriefers may use incompatible methodological approaches • Lack of preparation can lead to debriefers not working in harmony without a shared mental model of the learning objectives to be addressed • Potential for power struggle, domination, or disagreement among debriefers • Disagreement among debriefers regarding priorities and/or topics to be discussed (lack of a common plan) • Competition between debriefers to cover the points they care most about due to personal interest or professional bias in the case of an interprofessional simulation activity • One of the debriefers can remain silent and therefore cannot take on the role of co-debriefer • One debriefer is not allowing the expertise or strength of the other debriefer to be fully utilized • Debriefers may interrupt each other or talk too much giving participants little opportunity to express themselves • Both debriefers represent the same professional group and overlook participants from other professions • The use of two debriefers could be perceived as an excessive "educational force"

However, the presence of a co-debriefer also poses a number of issues and disadvantages that can lead to disastrous outcomes, especially if the two facilitators are not in sync and sufficiently trained to work together. Table 2.3 lists the benefits and disadvantages of a co-debriefing process.

2.10 Concluding Remarks

Debriefing is a critical component in the simulation-based health education process. It is very likely that any debriefing method can be effective when used appropriately and by experienced simulation facilitators. Furthermore, it is very likely that there is no "best" way to conduct a debriefing, but rather several methods from which simulation educators can choose, depending on the context of the simulation exercise they are conducting and their skills and preferences.

In all cases, using a well-structured debriefing allows the conversation to unfold in an orderly fashion, promotes efficient use of time, keeps the discussion on track, and focuses the conversation on important learning objectives. Without structure, the debriefing conversation risks degrading into a series of unfocused comments or observations.

The success of one debriefing technique over another strongly depends on the experience and competence of the debriefer, as well as on the experience and competence of the group of learners, and is certainly related to the type of scenario and simulation and its learning objectives.

References

1. Kolb, A. Y., & Kolb, D. A. (2009). The learning way: Meta-cognitive aspects of experiential learning. *Simulation and Gaming, 40*(3), 297–327.
2. Gardner, R. (2013). Introduction to debriefing. *Seminars in Perinatology, 37*(3), 166–174.
3. Raemer, D., Anderson, M., Cheng, A., Fanning, R., Nadkarni, V., & Savoldelli, G. (2011). Research regarding debriefing as part of the learning process. *Simulation in Healthcare, 6*(*Suppl*), S52–S57.
4. O'Donnell, J., Rodgers, D., Lee, W., Edelson, D., Haag, J., Hamilton, M., et al. (2009). *Structured and supported debriefing.* American Heart Association.
5. Rothgeb, M. K. (2008). Creating a nursing simulation laboratory: A literature review. *The Journal of Nursing Education, 47*(11), 489–494.
6. Weinstock, P. (2013). *Boston children's hospital simulator program, simulation instructor workshop. Personal communication.* Harvard University.
7. Kriz, W. C. (2010). A systemic-constructivist approach to the facilitation and debriefing of simulations and games. *Simulation and Gaming, 41*(5), 663–680.
8. Dieckmann, P., Molin Friis, S., Lippert, A., & Ostergaard, D. (2009). The art and science of debriefing in simulation: Ideal and practice. *Medical Teacher, 31*(7), e287–e294.
9. Motola, I., Devine, L. A., Chung, H. S., Sullivan, J. E., & Issenberg, S. B. (2013). Simulation in healthcare education: A best evidence practical guide. AMEE Guide No. 82. *The Medical Teacher, 35*(10), e1511–e1530.
10. Decker, S., Fey, M., Sideras, S., Caballero, S., Rockstraw, L. R., Boese, T., Franklin, A. E., Gloe, D., Lioce, L., Sando, C. R., Meakim, C., & Borum, J. C. (2013). Standards of best practice: Simulation standard VI: The debriefing process. *Clinical Simulation in Nursing, 9*(6 SUPPL), S26–S29.
11. Cheng, A., Eppich, W., Grant, V., Sherbino, J., Zendejas, B., & Cook, D. A. (2014). Debriefing for technology-enhanced simulation: A systematic review and meta-analysis. *Medical Education, 48*(7), 657–666.
12. De Vita, M. A., Schaefer, J., Lutz, J., Wang, H., & Dongilli, T. (2005). Improving medical emergency team (MET) performance using a novel curriculum and a computerized human patient simulator. *Quality and Safety in Health Care, 14*(5), 326–331.
13. Dine, C. J., Gersh, R. E., Leary, M., Riegel, B. J., Bellini, L. M., & Abella, B. S. (2008). Improving cardiopulmonary resuscitation quality and resuscitation training by combining audiovisual feedback and debriefing. *Critical Care Medicine, 36*(10), 2817–2822.
14. Falcone, R. A., Jr., Daugherty, M., Schweer, L., Patterson, M., Brown, R. L., & Garcia, V. F. (2008). Multidisciplinary pediatric trauma team training using high-fidelity trauma simulation. *Journal of Pediatric Surgery, 43*(6), 1065–1071.

15. Levett-Jones, T., & Lapkin, S. (2014). A systematic review of the effectiveness of simulation debriefing in health professional education. *Nurse Education Today, 34*(6), e58–e63.
16. Savoldelli, G. L., Naik, V. N., Park, J., Joo, H. S., Chow, R., & Hamstra, S. J. (2006). Value of debriefing during simulated crisis management: Oral versus video-assisted oral feedback. *Anesthesiology, 105*(2), 279–285.
17. Wayne, D. B., Didwania, A., Feinglass, J., Fudala, M. J., Barsuk, J. H., & McGaghie, W. C. (2008). Simulation-based education improves quality of care during cardiac arrest team responses at an academic teaching hospital: A case-control study. *Chest, 133*(1), 56–61.
18. Cheng, A., Morse, K. J., Rudolph, J., Arab, A. A., Runnacles, J., & Eppich, W. (2016). Learner-centered debriefing for health care simulation education: Lessons for faculty development. *Simulation in Healthcare, 11*(1), 32–40.
19. Miller, G. A. (1956). The magical number seven, plus or minus two: some limits on our capacity for processing information. *Psychol Rev, 63*(2), 81.
20. Choi, H. H., Van Merriënboer, J. J., & Paas, F. (2014). Effects of the physical environment on cognitive load and learning: Towards a new model of cognitive load. *Educational Psychology Review, 26*, 225–244.
21. Mitchell, A. M., Sakraida, T. J., & Kameg, K. (2003). Critical incident stress debriefing: Implications for best practice. *Disaster Management and Response, 1*(2), 46–51.
22. Der Sahakian, G., Alinier, G., Savoldelli, G., Oriot, D., Jaffrelot, M., & Lecomte, F. (2015). Setting conditions for productive debriefing. *Simulation and Gaming, 46*(2), 197–208.
23. Fanning, R. M., & Gaba, D. M. (2015). Debriefing. In D. M. Gaba, J. FishK, S. K. Howard, & A. R. Burden (Eds.), *Crisis management in anesthesiology* (2nd ed., pp. 65–78). Elsevier Saunders.
24. Fanning, R. M., & Gaba, D. M. (2007). The role of debriefing in simulation-based learning. *Simulation in Healthcare, 2*(2), 115–125.
25. Kolbe, M., Grande, B., & Spahn, D. R. (2015). Briefing and debriefing during simulation-based training and beyond: Content, structure, attitude and setting. *Best Practice and Research. Clinical Anaesthesiology, 29*(1), 87–96.
26. INACSL Standards Committee, McDermott, D. S., Ludlow, J., Horsley, E., & Meakim, C. (2021). Healthcare simulation standards of best practice TM prebriefing: Preparation and briefing. *Clinical Simulation in Nursing, 58*, 9–13.
27. Dieckmann, P., Gaba, D., & Rall, M. (2007). Deepening the theoretical foundations of patient simulation as social practice. *Simulation in Healthcare, 2*(3), 183–193.
28. Rudolph, J. W., Raemer, D. B., & Simon, R. (2014). Establishing a safe container for learning in simulation: The role of the presimulation briefing. *Simulation in Healthcare, 9*(6), 339–349.
29. Sawyer, T., Eppich, W., Brett-Fleegler, M., Grant, V., & Cheng, A. (2016). More than one way to debrief: A critical review of healthcare simulation debriefing methods. *Simulation in Healthcare, 11*(3), 209–217.
30. Brinko, K. T. (1993). The practice of giving feedback to improve teaching: What is effective? *The Journal of Higher Education, 64*, 574–593.
31. Telio, S., Ajjawi, R., & Regehr, G. (2015). The "educational alliance" as a framework for reconceptualizing feedback in medical education. *Academic Medicine, 90*(5), 609–614.
32. Lopreiato, J. O., Downing, D., Gammon, W., Lioce, L., Sittner, B., Slot, V., Spain, A. E., & The Terminology & Concepts Working Group (Eds.). (2016). *Healthcare simulation dictionary*. Agency for Healthcare Research and Quality AHRQ Publication. http://www.simmed.it/new/wp-content/uploads/2017/12/1624-simdictionary_ALL.pdf
33. Lefroy, J., Watling, C., Teunissen, P. W., & Brand, P. (2015). Guidelines: The do's, don'ts and don't knows of feedback for clinical education. *Perspectives on Medical Education, 4*, 284–299.
34. Parkes, J., Abercrombie, S., & McCarty, T. (2013). Feedback sandwiches affect perceptions but not performance. *Advances in Health Sciences Education: Theory and Practice, 18*(3), 397–407.

35. Boet, S., Bould, M. D., Bruppacher, H. R., Desjardins, F., Chandra, D. B., & Naik, V. N. (2011). Looking in the mirror: Self-debriefing versus instructor debriefing for simulated crises. *Critical Care Medicine, 39*(6), 1377–1381.
36. Smith-Jentsch, K. A., Cannon-Bowers, J. A., Tannenbaum, S. I., & Salas, E. (2008). Guided team self-correction: Impacts on team mental models, processes, and effectiveness. *Small Group Research, 39*(3), 303–327.
37. Fanning, R. M., Gaba, D. M. (2007). The role of debriefing in simulation-based learning. *Simulation in Healthcare* 2(2), 115–125.
38. Eppich, W., Cheng, A. (2015). Promoting Excellence and Reflective Learning in Simulation (PEARLS): development and rationale for a blended approach to health care simulation debriefing. *Simulation in Healthcare, 10*(2), 106–115.
39. O'Brien, C., Leeman, K., Roussin, C., Casey, D., Grandinetti, T., & Lindamood, K. (2017, June 1–3). *Using plus-delta-plus human factors debriefing to bridge simulation and clinical environments.* In International Pediatric Simulation Symposia and Workshop (IPSSW), Boston, MA.
40. Eppich, W., & Cheng, A. (2015). Promoting Excellence and Reflective Learning in Simulation (PEARLS): Development and rationale for a blended approach to health care simulation debriefing. *Simulation in Healthcare, 10*(2), 106–115.
41. Rudolph, J. W., Simon, R., Dufresne, R. L., & Raemer, D. B. (2006). There's no such thing as "nonjudgmental" debriefing: A theory and method for debriefing with good judgment. *Simulation in Healthcare, 1*(1), 49–55.
42. Colman, N., Dalpiaz, A., Walter, S., Chambers, M. S., & Hebbar, K. B. (2020). SAFEE: A debriefing tool to identify latent conditions in simulation-based hospital design testing. *Advances in Simulation, 5*, 14.

Effective Communication for Strategic Change

Communication is not what we say, but what reaches others.

Thorsten Havener

The real voyage of discovery consists, not in seeking new landscapes, but in having new eyes.

Marcel Proust

3.1 Introduction

"One cannot not communicate" is the first axiom of human communication [1]. Interpersonal communication occurs on multiple levels, including verbal and non-verbal, as all behavior is a form of communication and has a communication value that significantly contributes to our experience and perception of the word. Even an attempt to avoid conversation—for example, through silence—nonetheless communicates the sender's intent and feeling to the receiver. If this indeed is the case, we influence our interlocutor whether we like it or not or pay attention to it.[1] Still, we can choose whether to do so casually or strategically.

Knowing how to communicate effectively means, from a strategic perspective, setting the tone for a trust relationship and to evoke sensation, overcome resistance, and produce change. It also serves the function of helping professionals define the problem they are working on.

Inevitable in any change-based relationship or context is—in fact—the implicit paradoxical assertion by those seeking help to "change me without changing me." If we consider the fact that most individuals or extended human systems tend to resist any change that might alter their equilibrium—even when pathological or dysfunctional—then professionals must consider the use of the dialogue as an instrument of persuasion. With the words of Epicurus, "one should not violate nature but try to persuade it."

However, while trying to persuade someone, people commonly focus on the content of their argument (*what* to say), not adequately thinking about *how* to say it, and even less about the importance of listening before speaking. So, they often find themselves arguing, trying in vain to convince others of their opinions—but most of

---

[1] The rule states that 7% of meaning is communicated through spoken word, 38% through tone of voice, and 55% through body language [2].

© The Author(s), under exclusive license to Springer Nature
Switzerland AG 2022
G. Capogna et al., *Strategic Debriefing for Advanced Simulation*,
https://doi.org/10.1007/978-3-031-06104-2_3

the time remaining frustrated or with the feeling that the other is unreasonable. Even while listening, people generally do it intending to respond rather than understanding. The subtle self-deception according to which there is only one "right and true" representation of how things are precludes people from seeing that there is not a single true reality, but many realities depending on the individuals' points of view.

From a constructivist point of view [3] our perceptions, behaviors, and interactions essentially construct the world we inhabit, and once created, this gives us a sense of stability and illusion of order and control. Therefore, the world would be an outcome of our perceptions, and there would be no definitive version of things, even if we feel it to be so. This is why the use of belief in which logical-rational explanations are employed to bring the other to recognize our arguments is often unsuccessful and may even appear provocative or unpleasant to the interlocutor—thus destroying the opportunities which we are looking to create.

Persuading, or rather "gently leading to oneself," is a communicative process that guides the interlocutor in a soothing way and without forcing them to accept others' theses starting from their point of view. The persuasion path is never opposed to the convictions or beliefs of the other but respects and uses them, thus allowing to circumvent the individual's natural resistance to change.

As William James, the first great modern psychologist, stated: "genius is nothing other than the ability to perceive things from a non-ordinary perspective."

It is no coincidence that all the greatest scientists in history, from Archimedes to Edison, have made extensive use of non-ordinary logic to increase their ability to invent.

Logic can be seen as the method by which humans apply their knowledge, solve problems, and reach objectives, and it is therefore the bridge between theory and practice [4].

The Aristotelian ordinary logic—which informs rational thinking and relies on premises of "true/false," "no third value," and the principles of "non-contradiction"— adheres to the belief in the primacy of coherence and congruence to cause and affect thinking. But "for a human being to be in contradiction is a rule, not an exception" [5], and we should refuse any theory that claims to describe how reality works and that would prescribe change in a rational manner. This does not mean that ordinary logic is wrong or is a useless invention. However, if it's correct and functional when applied to natural linear phenomenon, it's completely incorrect when used with self-referential recursive phenomena like most humans' problems. To effectively intervene on them, following the Hippocratic axiom "similia similibus curantur" (like is cured by like), we need a different logic that follows their structure and that is able to reorient their direction toward a functional management.

Non-ordinary logics—the logic of belief, paradox, and contradiction—allow us to manage resistance and construct interventions that help us adapt the solution to the problem we are working on. It also helps us avoid being trapped by ideology or theory and to handle human ambivalence [4].

In the same way, it is possible to discover new and efficient solutions to a given problem that were previously invisible by formulating and trying to respond to particular forms of questioning designed to create "alternatives" that lead one to assume diverse perspectives about the problem.

With the recent discovery of mirror neurons [6, 7], even modern neurosciences show that when two individuals come into contact and "tune in," the same areas of the brain are activated in a sort of identification at the neural level that triggers the same emotions. This shows that the human mind and brain have evolved and specialized precisely by increasingly refined forms of communicative exchanges and further highlights the importance of studying the type of language best suited to induce change.

3.2 Knowing to See by Learning How to Act: Theory Informing the Brief Strategic Approach

The brief strategic approach represents a major shift from the ordinary ways of defining and intervening on humans' difficulties that leads to a more function-based knowledge and practice, underpinned by the notion of *attempted solution*.

This was first introduced by the team at Mental Research Institute (MRI) in Palo Alto [8, 9] and later evolved into the construct of the *perceptive-reactive system* developed by Giorgio Nardone [10]. It embodies the spontaneous reactions and behaviors of a person in facing difficulties and getting rid of a problem in the relationship with him/herself, others, and the world. If the solution works, then the problem is solved, but if it does not, and the unhelpful solutions are applied and reapplied, they usually end up becoming rigid, redundant, dysfunctional models of interaction with the reality that complicate rather than solve the problem. These circuits work in such a way that when the organism faces situations that are the same or similar to those encountered in the past, reactions are spontaneously activated independently of cognitive reasons and expectations [11]. So, when operating on a problem and observing the attempted solutions of a person, the professional can see them as a reducer of complexity that can assist in creating a practical, rigorous, and innovative diagnostic framework for treatment that follows the same non-ordinary logic that underlies the problem at hand and thereby allows the solution that arises to be more likely to adhere to the system from which they arose.

Therefore, to substitute the dysfunctional attempted solutions with a more functional one, it is necessary to study the mental, emotional, and relational "traps" in which people might find themselves. At the same time, to get to know a problem through its solution, it is crucial to identify the strategic levers of change (the rules of the ongoing game) [12–14].

As Gregory Bateson [15] stated, all we can do is to observe *how* a system functions and how we can help it function better by intervening on it and observing the outcome of our intervention to know how to intervene better. If the effect creates positive change, then we can continue; if it does not, then we alter our strategy or overturn our theory of the problem [15]. This process helps us avoid what Karl Popper called self-sealing prepositions—those kinds of ideas that essentially prove their validity [16].

"Knowing through changing" therefore becomes the operative construct of strategic intervention, because it is through changing the perception and the vision of a person that we can lead them to discover new, solution-orientated ways of perceiving and managing their problems and difficulties [17, 18]. As von Foerster echoes, "if you desire to see, learn how to act" [19].

Moreover, Franz Alexander sustains that "intellectual insight alone is not sufficient" and that individuals need to go through a *corrective emotional experience* to feel differently and be freed from their constraining sensations, perceptions, and reactions [20].

This idea collides with the assumption that to change a problematic behavior, one should primarily change the person's way of thinking via the use of reasoning and indicative, descriptive, explanatory, confrontational, and interpretative language. After all, the question of *why* a problem exists in the first place is often more of interest of the professional than the client, who usually looks at how to get rid of the problem [21].

The use of a suggestive, evocative, performative, and injunctive language— instead—offers the person new ways to act as it leads people to experience something that rational explanations cannot provide by directly stimulating the most archaic part of the human brain (paleoencephalon).

Thomas Aquinas said that "nihil est in intellectu quod non sit prius in sensu" (nothing is in the intellect that was not first in the senses). Accordingly, this statement is being evermore confirmed by neurosciences, which postulate that 80% of our brain activities take place below the level of consciousness [22]. Rational components would therefore only partially be able to regulate emotions, which respond to concrete experiences, and in turn, produce important effects on a conscious level (cerebrum). Emotions are skills without understanding, and any attempt to control them (i.e., pleasure or fear) based on rational processes would collapse on itself (paradoxical effect) generating dysfunctional responses [23].

Thus, changing the point of view represents an illuminating joint discovery of two individuals through a dialogue purposely designed to lead the person to have real or elicited experiences that—eluding the control of the Cerebrum—come directly to the paleoencephalon and cannot be carried out at a cognitive level.

3.3 The Structure of the Strategic Dialogue

The roots of the word dialogue come from the Greek words *dia* (through) and *logos* ("word" or "meaning"). A dialogue is, therefore, a flow of meaning. But it is more than this. In the most ancient connotation of the word, *logos* meant "to gather together" and suggests a conversation in which people think together in the relationship. Thinking together implies that you no longer take your position as final but listen to possibilities that might not otherwise have occurred as a result of simply being in a relationship with others [16].

Protagoras—one of the most important sophists—was the first who made use of the dialogue as a persuasive technique. He designed the so-called Eristic dialogue (*eristikè tèchne*—the art of argumentation), consisting of putting forward questions structured in a specific successive order to elicit responses from the interlocutor that would follow the desired direction of the persuader. By doing so, confrontations are avoided, and the sender can persuade the receiver of his/her thesis [24] but making them feel responsible for the discovery.

The strategic dialog is based on a theory of radical constructivism, which postulates that problems that occur in human systems are a product of our interaction, between ourselves, the others, and our unique and self-invented reality. Because humans are closed systems, and since they rely on their internal central nervous system to interpret all the information coming from the outside world, they can never have pure knowledge of the "real" world—but they contaminate that which they observe [3].

Through seemingly simple and thus disarming communication techniques including *questions with the illusion of an alternative, reframing, and paraphrasing*, as well as the use of *evocative language* (i.e., metaphors, analogies aphorisms, and anecdotes), the strategic dialog leads the person to assume a diverse perspective and to discover the solution to their problem in a sort of natural and spontaneous evolution that overcomes the usual resistance to change and makes them feel the main protagonist and artifact of the therapeutic change.

By doing so, change can be produced from the first encounter, which becomes a true change-inducing intervention phase. In this way, rather than only guiding the professional in assessing the "true" nature of the problem to be solved, the dialogue is used to induce the client's reactions to change and bring to light their resources that have been jammed by the previous rigid yet dysfunctional perceptive reactive system.

Then, the therapeutic prescriptions became the spontaneous evolution of the dialogue, and not just an assignment bearing no obvious relation to the presenting problem, as clients sometimes might perceive (Fig. 3.1).

Fig. 3.1 Sequence of the strategic dialogue [25]

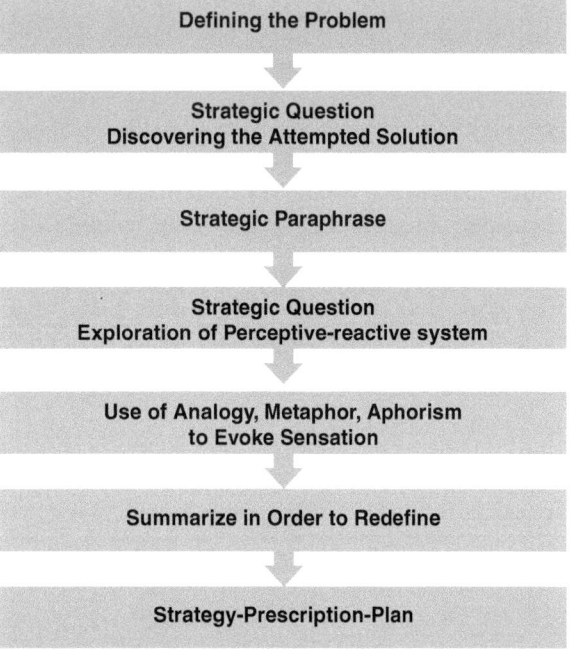

Defining the Problem

Strategic Question
Discovering the Attempted Solution

Strategic Paraphrase

Strategic Question
Exploration of Perceptive-reactive system

Use of Analogy, Metaphor, Aphorism
to Evoke Sensation

Summarize in Order to Redefine

Strategy-Prescription-Plan

3.3.1   Use of the Strategic Questioning

To understand the other's point of view and *defining the problem* properly, the initial step is to let them argue. To this aim, the conversation can be started with an *open question* (i.e., "What is the problem that brings you here?", "Can you explain your situation to me?", "I would like to understand better what you feel," etc.).

Then, the dialog moves from the general to the specific. The questions are no longer open-ended but are altered in their interrogative form to begin to include *discriminating* and *intervening/restructuring questions with an illusion of alternatives*.

This technique represents one of the most elegant forms of injunction [10, 26]. Questions are structured in such a way that they hold two possible answers, among which the person replies by taking up the one that best fits their situation. As the dialog proceeds, the sequence of questions is structured as a sort of funnel that starts with general questions and gradually narrows down in a spiral fashion and builds upon answers that reveal potentially critical aspects of the particular emerging situation.

Questions are not pre-established, but—to be real therapeutic instruments and vehicles of change—they are tailored to the logic of the interlocutor and constructed to call and reorient the perceptions and reactions of the subject to more functional ones [16] (Fig. 3.2).

Discriminating questions focus on the concrete interaction between the person and their problematic reality, i.e., on their failed attempts to manage it (*reactions*) and on the perception that feeds them to detect the most relevant characteristics of the individuals' perceptive-reactive system.

These allow for the asking of information about the problem across space (*where*, i.e., does it happen only at home or also in other places?), time (*when*, i.e., does it happen always or only at certain times of the day?), mechanisms of action (*how*, i.e., does it happen spontaneously, or is it stimulated by something? "When faced with problematic situations, do you tend to run away or confront them directly?" In these situations what do you do? Do you *wait* or *intervene*?), and people involved (*who*, i.e., does it only affect you or also other people? "Do you face the situation alone or ask someone for help?").

Still, strategic questions are not only meant to help the professional to learn how the problem functions but represent a very powerful intervention tool. Once the professional has gained enough information about how the problem functions based on the individuals' dysfunctional attempted solutions, restructuring questions (i.e., when you tried, did anything change, or did everything remain unchanged? After having done [something], did you feel better or worse? By avoiding, did your fear diminished or increased over the years?) are used to evoke new ways of feeling and reacting. The individuals' attempts to solve the situation, from being useful, start to be spontaneously perceived as problematic, and gradually the person feels the

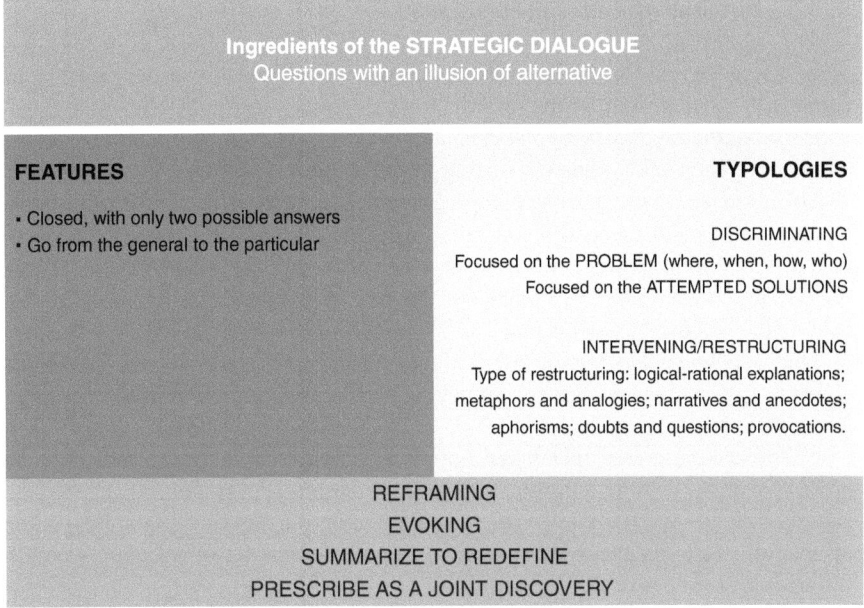

Fig. 3.2 Ingredients of the strategic dialogue

perspective proposed by the persuader as a conjunct discovery. This allows to completely bypass resistance to change and to achieve a true corrective emotional experience [20] based on which the subject can only change their previous mental and behavioral patterns.

With the words of Pascal: "people are generally better persuaded by the reasons which they have themselves discovered than by those which come into the mind of others" [27].

At the same time, an emotionally positive relationship that amplifies the collaboration and the subject's expectations over the therapy is established.

While asking, it is important that the professional's "nonverbal" also communicate listening and attention: the posture must be relaxed, the gaze floating on the face and the course of the other, all accompanied by mimic nods of agreement that communicate that we are listening and understanding—and which also trigger similar nonverbal responses in the interlocutor in reciprocity that further contributes to the creation of a good therapeutic relationship and leads to the possibility of a final agreement.

This is of great importance since, like Hubble reminds us, a strong therapeutic relationship is responsible for over 70% of the change achieved during treatment [28].

3.3.2   Reframing and Paraphrases

After a sequence of two or three strategic questions, the professional provides the client with a redefinition of the information gathered to verify the understanding of their words (the diagnostic hypothesis) and to send back to them a reframed version of what has been said—thus facilitating the change process.

The clinician might start the paraphrase with "Correct me if I'm wrong ..." and/ or "If I understand correctly, you're telling me ..."—thus assuming a one-down position that communicates an eagerness to understand the client's point of view without judgment, increases collaboration, and makes the person feel as if they are leading the discovery process.

The acceptance of a paraphrase is also a subtle form of self-persuasion. On the contrary, if the person does not accept it, the professional will be able to accordingly adjust their questioning.

Effective paraphrasing is not just limited to verification, but it can also allow the professional to re-punctuate the sequence of events. Punctuation is a powerful aspect of the axiom of human communication in organizing the individuals' casual attribution of the problem [1] since—as Pascal reminds us—"the same words in different sequence give different results."

For example, the professional might ask "If I understand correctly, but you correct me if I'm wrong, after having done [something], you feel worse, rather than better ..."

By doing so, the person does not feel disqualified but rather gratified, under-stood, and emotionally reinforced, besides further acknowledging how the problem functions and how they can best manage it.

3.3.3   Evoking Sensation

Then, the professional can further reinforce the effects of what has already been reached using metaphors, aphorisms, anecdotes, or concrete argumentation using non-ordinary logic. After all, "a picture is worth a thousand words."

Nardone and Watzlavick [10] sustain that the use of analogical and figurative language reduces resistance to change since the persons' opinion and behavior are not criticized, but the message gets through in disguise, in a manner of speaking. Suggestions must directly target the person perceptive modalities which underlie their dysfunctional reactions to the problem, communicative style, and personal characteristics and be embedded in a story or communicated through metaphor in such a way the subject is not directly involved, but their evocative power counteracts the person's self-reinforcing conceptions or behaviors.

This observation is directly related to Bandler and Grinder's [29, 30] idea that people deal with problems in different sensory channels. They maintain that a problem framed in one channel will facilitate its resolution, while dealing with it in another channel would leave the person at an impasse [29, 30].

Through its form of "non-directive directivity," the strategic dialogue works on four basic levels simultaneously: perception, emotion, behavior, and cognition.

Thus, analogical language can be reoriented at either creating aversion toward the attitudes or behaviors to be interrupted or changed (attempted solutions) or at enhancing the client's reactions that need to be stimulated or increased to make the person feel the necessity and unavoidability of change.

3.3.4 Summarize to Redefine

Once with the phase of inquiry-discovery a new perspective has been induced, the professional proceeds to summarize and frame what has been achieved to consolidate the accomplished persuasive process. This summarizing aims to provide a final redefinition of the jointly achieved discoveries, which is offered as an articulated sequence of the client's answers and pinpoint the agreement which has been earlier achieved. This maneuver, as a sort of hyper-paraphrases, consolidates and increases all the previously induced effects, making them converge toward changes required for unblocking the individuals' resources.

3.4   Prescription as an Outcome

Only when the person has been engaged, their problem defined, and perspective qualified can the professional move to the prescription phase. Thanks to the dialogue achievement, the person will be willing to accept suggestions or even direct prescriptions regarding the stratagems to be carried out.

Hence, prescriptions not only become acceptable but also inevitable, seeing as they are the direct effect of what both people have previously accomplished and agreed upon.

The use of hypnotic communication techniques without trance resulting from the work of the medical hypnotist Milton Erikson (i.e., prosody or pausing for emphasis and focus, suggestive and strategic repetitions of the prescription and the introduction of redundancy) and performative language, also the timing of the prescription, all increment the persuasive effect that helps enhance the client's motivation to follow the therapeutic indications [26].

As Henrik Ibsen first said, "a thousand words leave not the same deep impression as does a single deed."

Notably, ending the session with a prescription means the client exits the session with the "sound" ringing in their ears, and so it should not be interrupted with too much conversational clutter after the session concludes. John Weakland used to say that the therapy starts when the client sat down and ends when she/he stood up.

3.5   Conclusion

The evolution of therapeutic communication has transformed the style of the first encounter into a true intervention. Just like a wise strategist, the clinician makes use of subtle communicative maneuvers to bypass the individuals' natural resistance to change and to guide them not to "understand" but to "feel" their problem differently. In this way, the interlocutor gets more easily persuaded of what she/he has come to discover while feeling the main protagonist of the scene.

Therefore, the therapeutic power of the strategic dialogue resides in its "surprising essentiality" or, better, in guiding persons entrapped in their problems to get to know how to solve them in a sort of natural and spontaneous evolution throughout a therapeutic conversation. In the wake of this, *maximum results are achieved with minimum effort.*

References

1. Watzlawick, P., Bavelas, J. B., & Jackson, D. D. (1967). *Pragmatics of human communication: A study of interactional patterns, pathologies, and paradoxes.* Norton.
2. Mehrabian, A. (1971). *Silent Messages: Implicit Communication of Emotions and Attitudes.* Belmont, California: Wadsworth Publishing.
3. Watzlawick, P. (1984). *The invented reality.* Norton.
4. Nardone, G., & Balbi, E. (2008). *The logic of therapeutic change: Fitting strategies to pathologies.* Routledge.
5. Bateson, G. (2002). *Mind and nature: A necessary unity.* Hampton Press.
6. Gallese, V., Fadiga, L., Fogassi, L., & Rizzolatti, G. (1996). Action recognition in the premotor cortex. [Research Support, Non-U.S. Gov't]. *Brain, 119*(Pt 2), 593–609. https://doi.org/10.1093/brain/119.2.593
7. Rizzolatti, G. (2005). The mirror neuron system and its function in humans. [Research Support, Non-U.S. Gov't]. *Anatomy and Embryology (Berl), 210*(5–6), 419–421. https://doi.org/10.1007/s00429-005-0039-z
8. Watzlawick, P., Weakland, J., & Fisch, R. (1974). *Change: Principles of problem formation and problem solution.* Norton.
9. Weakland, J. H., Fisch, R., Watzlawick, P., & Bordin, A. M. (1974). Brief therapy: Focused problem resolution. *Family Process, 13*(2), 141–168.
10. Nardone, G., & Watzlawick, P. (2005). *Brief strategic therapy. Philosophy, techniques, and research.* Jason Aronson.
11. Pietrabissa, G., Manzoni, G. M., Rossi, A., & Castelnuovo, G. (2017). The MOTIV-HEART study: A prospective, randomized, single-blind pilot study of brief strategic therapy and motivational interviewing among cardiac rehabilitation patients. *Frontiers in Psychology, 8*, 83. https://doi.org/10.3389/fpsyg.2017.00083
12. Jackson, J. B., Pietrabissa, G., Rossi, A., Manzoni, G. M., & Castelnuovo, G. (2018). Brief strategic therapy and cognitive behavioral therapy for women with binge eating disorder and comorbid obesity: A randomized clinical trial one-year follow-up. [Randomized Controlled Trial]. *Journal of Consulting and Clinical Psychology, 86*(8), 688–701. https://doi.org/10.1037/ccp0000313
13. Nardone, G., & Watzlawick, P. (1993). *The art of change.* Jossey-Bass.
14. Pietrabissa, G., Manzoni, G. M., Gibson, P., Boardman, D., Gori, A., & Castelnuovo, G. (2016). Brief strategic therapy for obsessive-compulsive disorder: A clinical and research protocol of a

one-group observational study. [Observational Study]. *BMJ Open, 6*(3), e009118. https://doi.org/10.1136/bmjopen-2015-009118

15. Bateson, G. (1972). *Steps to an ecology of mind*. Ballantine.
16. Nardone, G., & Salvini, A. (2007). *The strategic dialogue: Rendering the diagnostic interview a real therapeutic intervention* (1st ed.). Routledge.
17. Nardone, G., & Portelli, C. (2005). *Knowing through changing: The evolution of brief strategic therapy*. Crown.
18. Pietrabissa, G., Castelnuovo, G., Jackson, J. B., Rossi, A., Manzoni, G. M., & Gibson, P. (2019). Brief strategic therapy for bulimia nervosa and binge eating disorder: A clinical and research protocol. *Frontiers in Psychology, 10*, 373. https://doi.org/10.3389/fpsyg.2019.00373
19. von Foerster, H., von Glasersfeld, E., Hejl, P. M., Schmidt, S. J., & Paul Watzlawick, P. (1997). *Einführung In Den Konstruktivismus*. Piper.
20. Alexander, F., & French, T. M. (1946). *Psychoanalytic therapy*. Ronald Press.
21. Pietrabissa, G., Rozzoni, F., Liguori, F., Cerruto, A., Giusti, E. M., Malfatto, G., et al. (2020). The brief strategic treatment of cardiophobia: A clinical case study. *Journal of Contemporary Psychotherapy*. https://doi.org/10.1007/s10879-020-09479-z
22. Koch, C. (2012). *Consciousness: Confessions of a romantic reductionist*. The MIT Press.
23. Nardone, G. (2015). *La nobile arte della persuasione. La magia delle parole e dei gesti*. Ponte alle Grazie.
24. Volpi, F. (1991). *L'arte di ottenere ragione*. Adelphi.
25. Gibson, P. (2019). *Advances in effective brief psychotherapy: Strategies relationships communication*. Lettertec Publishing.
26. Loriedo, C., Nardone, G., Watzlawick, P., & Zeig, J. K. (2002). *Strategie e stratagemmi nella psicoterapia. Tecniche ipnotiche e non ipnotiche per la soluzione, in tempi brevi, di problemi complessi*. Franco Angeli.
27. Pascal, B. (1995). *Pensées*. Penguin Classics.
28. Hubble, M., Miller, B., & Duncan, S. (1999). *The heart and soul of change: What works in therapy*. American Psychological Association.
29. Bandler, R., & Grinder, J. (1975). *The structure of magic* (Vol. I). Science and Behavior Books.
30. Grinder, J., & Bandler, R. (1976). *The structure of magic* (Vol. II). Science and Behavior Books.

Strategic Debriefing: A Corrective Emotional Experience

4

Before convincing the intellect, one must touch the heart.

Blaise Pascal

"No one can understand something well and make it his own when he has learned it from another than when he has learned it himself." This sentence by Descartes sums up the essence of simulation, which considers learning *by doing* as an essential and necessary factor for adult learning. It is not enough to "know" and "know how to do," but this must be integrated with "knowing how to communicate." However, it is well-known that reality is the experience of our perceptions that strongly interact with our emotions.

For this reason, the EESOA Simulation Centre-Debriefers Training School has applied to debriefing the principles of dialogue and strategic *problem-solving* and brief strategic therapy [1] built on the basis of the theoretical formulations and applications of the theories of Paul Watzlawick and Giorgio Nardone [2–6] and using the models of the Strategic Therapy Centre of Arezzo, founded and directed by Giorgio Nardone.

The strategic model deals with the way in which man perceives and manages his own reality through communication with himself, others, and the world, transforming it from dysfunctional to functional, in order to be able to operate on it. The strategic dialogue, alternating analogical and digital language, using metaphors and paraphrases, leads the participant to live a corrective emotional experience, which is the first cause of change. The structure of strategic dialogue is based on the use of the illusion of alternatives, restructuring paraphrases, evocation of feelings, and summarizing redefinitions, until the joint discovery that leads to change. This dialogue can be used in the debriefing after the scenario which, while maintaining its typical phases (reaction, description, analysis and application), is enriched by a deeper and more persistent inquiry whose effectiveness is confirmed in the application phase, in the student's discovery of concrete and actionable goals, agents of clinical and behavioral change in the field.

G. Capogna et al., *Strategic Debriefing for Advanced Simulation*, https://doi.org/10.1007/978-3-031-06104-2_4

4.1   Emotions and Simulation

Doctors have too often cultivated the illusion of a purely rational and objective knowledge, uncontaminated by passions and feelings, based on the myth that considers cognitive processes as "superior" to the world of emotions. Even as students, people are often trained to "not get caught up in emotions" in order to better focus on patients, and it is generally believed that emotions are something independent of rational thought and are experienced exclusively at a visceral level or can be controlled by reason.

Emotions can be considered as part of one's information processing system, a kind of thinking alongside conscious thought. They constitute a subconscious, rapid, and global evaluation of the situation or event you are experiencing. This evaluation is very rapid and automatic and processes much more information than conscious perception. If the emotional and cognitive evaluations of situations are different from each other, i.e., our mind and instincts tell us different things, we tend to be confused. The reason is that emotions use different (and faster) neural pathways than conscious reasoning, and as soon as they are perceived, they can be further processed like any other perceived data and thus provide the basis for our decision-making processes. For example, a decision may be delayed because we want to avoid the feeling of failure, or, conversely, an action may be taken only because we anticipate the feeling of success.

Generally, in situations where cognitive resources are overstretched or are in some way inadequate, such as in medical emergencies, humans let emotions guide their behavior [7]. For example, on an emotional basis, quick and risky solutions may be chosen without thought, or problems are oversimplified and solutions considered satisfactory just because they "feel good." This can lead to poor decisions, if the subconscious goal becomes maintaining one's sense of competence and self-esteem, or to an escape from negative emotions rather than doing the best thing for that patient at that particular time.

Daily experience shows that the way in which a task is performed depends very much on the emotional state of the operator (e.g., the same thing done calmly or angrily may seem completely different). An "angry" way of acting will in fact be characterized by greater excitement, less cognitive evaluation of actions, poor planning, and incomplete reflection on possible ways of operating.

Certain feelings (e.g., anger, joy, fear) may act as a stimulus. This phenomenon, known as nonspecific sympathetic syndrome, increases readiness to explore the environment and prepare for action. The senses are alert, and muscle tone, blood pressure, heart rate, and breathing rate increase. Other feelings, however, such as sadness or despair, decrease the level of activation.

Depending on the emotional situation, a cognitive process (e.g., perception, thought) may take place with varying degrees of resolution with respect to normal conditions and, therefore, with different precision. By "degree of resolution" we mean the level of differentiation and discrimination between the cognitive and perceptual dimensions. One can assess facts in an accurate and minute way, or simply consider the salient aspects of a situation. The effectiveness with which environmental factors are broken down and considered in decision-making depends on emotions (through the level of activation), the importance of the situation, and time constraints (subjectively assessed). For the clinician, the consequence is that emotions may condition the diagnostic-decisional behavior with respect to the patient, contributing to the development of a picture of the situation that is either too superficial or too detailed and all encompassing. For example, in the case of a particular repulsion to a task, the degree of resolution will be diminished and the objective perception of reality only rough, so that the performance is likely to be superficial.

Strong arousal increases the threshold of selective attention, above which an alternative motivation succeeds in replacing a main motivation and becomes, in turn, the major driver of action. If the selective attention threshold is high, people will tend to adhere more steadily to their task, without becoming distracted. If this threshold increases further, it may reach a level at which it is no longer possible to react to external stimuli (e.g., the alarm of a monitor or the calls of other team members who are unable to penetrate this "wall of concentration").

Conversely, when people feel a sense of powerlessness, or have the impression that they are not up to a problem, the selection threshold for action is decreased. In the hope of bringing about some change, they will try whatever comes to mind.

Emotions thus influence the extent to which attention is focused on external events or on internal cognitive processes (reflection, planning). In this way, emotions have a primary impact in determining how much a person's behavior is event-driven or follows cognitive processes. For example, angry or fearful people will focus on the initial stimulus and how to get rid of it, instead of focusing their thinking on the main problem, raising their voice to others instead of asking the right questions.

Simulation teaches both technical *skills*, i.e., the knowledge, skill, and ability to perform a specific medical task, for example, inserting a chest drain or performing a physical examination, and *non-technical* or behavioral skills, i.e., communication skills, *leadership*, teamwork, situational awareness, decision-making, resource management, safe practices, and minimizing adverse events.

The awareness that emotions can strongly regulate and condition human behavior has led our Training School to define a further skill to be added to the previous ones traditionally taught with simulation: *emotional skills*.

Aware that the ability to manage emotions is beyond the ordinary skills of a debriefer, even a strategic one, we nevertheless believe that the acquisition of some basic knowledge about them can help the debriefer himself in his educational task and complement his activities of facilitating the discussion after a simulation.

The source of emotions can be analyzed, and their intensity can be changed through familiarization with their meaning and by learning how to incorporate emotional data into action. During a medical emergency, whether real or simulated, fear and pain, anger, and pleasure can take dysfunctional forms that limit performance. The simulation with a strategic approach that we have introduced initiates a reflection on how to "tame" emotions and then recognize them, transforming limitations into extremely powerful resources.

The first crucial moment in which the debriefer addresses the emotions of the scenario participants is the reaction phase. This phase, in addition to helping the trainees to decompress and get out of the role they played during the scenario, is very useful for the debriefer to understand the emotional state of each of the trainees, which will inevitably, if not handled appropriately, reflect negatively in turn on the debriefing discussion and the learning itself.

The strategic model we propose deepens this phase (see paragraph 4.2), usually superficially confined to the simple "venting of the students," making it a real first phase of emotional deepening, preliminary to the debriefing itself.

4.2   How to Help Learners Deal with the Emotions Felt During the Scenario

It is well-known that a simulated scenario induces the same emotions as a real clinical scenario and that emotions are activated through subcortical non-conscious recognition, which bypasses conscious control itself, inducing unconscious emotional reactions that often guide the actions of the trainees during the scenario. There are four primary emotions, to which all others can be traced: anger, pleasure, fear, and pain: they are the levers of most of our changes and our performance, so they must be known and managed by the debriefer, so that he can help his students do the same.

In the reaction phase, with the strategic approach we propose, the participant acquires the inner awareness of the real sensation/deep basic emotion that the scenario has aroused: evoking it, recognizing it, and becoming aware of it, he can let it flow, follow its flow, and, with the help of the strategic debriefer, use it in a constructive way.

The ways proposed and usually used to manage emotions are basically three: let them vent, control, or condition them (for more details, see [8]). It is commonplace that releasing accumulated emotional tension frees us from stress. However, if we try to vent our anger for a wrong suffered with someone willing to listen to us, not only is the anger not reduced, but it increases, because it is confirmed by the listener's acceptance of the argument. The same thing happens with fear: talking about it in order to reduce anxiety, we end up exacerbating it, and if our interlocutor tries to support us, it becomes more intense, confirming our inability to manage this emotion. Venting one's pain can generate the effect of making us feel important to the other who cares for us, attracting more attention to us, and so we end up complacent in the pain instead of coming out of it. Venting a pleasure to which we no longer wish to be subjugated results in the more we talk about it, the more we enjoy it, and we end up increasing our irreversible attraction to what we wanted to avoid.

Although we know that emotions escape rational logic, their control is often suggested as a method for their management. "In the face of fear the arguments of reason are as ineffective as the subterfuges of hope." This phrase by Cioran expresses well the fact that fear, like the other three basic emotions, being a fundamentally irrational emotional reaction, cannot be managed with the tools of logic.

In experimental psychology, attempts have also been made to manage emotions with conditioning, through negative or positive reinforcement, constructing conditioned reflexes, but with little success in application except to very specific cases.

To oppose emotions would therefore be like pretending to want to stop the flood of a river by pushing the water with your hands. The first important step, therefore, in learning to manage emotions is to "allow" them, or to avoid opposing them, because allowing them to be expressed makes them flow naturally without exacerbating or transforming them, as happens when we try to repress or control them. In practice, go with the flow to use the force in a constructive way, and consider the emotions as the driving force of change, and then use them as such. But to manage emotions, we must use their language, which is not that of logical and rational explanations but that of suggestions, evocations, and concrete experiences.

As in real life, even during the simulated scenario, fear is the basic emotion that occurs most frequently, although it is often reported superficially and masked, for example, by anxiety (performance), by prejudice (I do something because I'm afraid that something else will happen to me or to the patient), or by insecurity (fear of making a mistake). Faced with fear, we are paralyzed and often astonished by the speed with which it sets in and conditions our actions subtly, without our permission. The debriefer, through strategic dialogue, can help the student observe how fear should be considered as a resource and not a limitation. In fact, fear is a mechanism that, within physiological limits, is positive and, indeed, helps overcome and resolve stressful situations. It is only when it exceeds a certain threshold that, becoming panic or a chronic dysfunctional reaction, can it have negative consequences on performance.

It is therefore not a matter of repressing or inhibiting the emotional response, but of regulating it by managing the way we perceive what triggers it.

In terms of managing perceptions, which in turn activate emotions, the first step is learning to broaden the point of view from which you see things.

The debriefer should be able to take the pupil's perceptual perspective to the point where even that which disturbs him in his reasoning is reasonable and justifiable. Only then, and certainly after much practice, will he be able to add his own point of view, broadening the pupil's view and thus persuading him that there is also a possible different perception.

4.3 Descriptive Phase

Similar to the descriptive phase of the standard debriefing, strategic debriefing also explores in this phase what happened during the scenario through the eyes and narrative of the participants.

The description process consists of leading the group through an "agreed description" of the scenario that has just ended. This should be done on an action-by-action basis, limiting the discussion to the statement of facts and avoiding emotions and comments. The typical question in this phase is "What did you see?" or "What happened?" The focus should remain on creating a shared understanding of what actually happened in the scenario. This ensures that scenario participants do not feel under attack and that a safe learning environment is maintained. At the end of the descriptive phase, in accordance with the strategic dialogue, the debriefer uses the technique of paraphrasing (see below) to summarize what happened in a non-judgmental way and to establish agreement among the participants about what happened and what was experienced and perceived by individuals and the group itself. In this way, already in this preliminary phase, the debriefer can explore and begin to define the experiences and perceptions of each of his or her students, which will most likely have conditioned the behavior during the scenario that will be explored in the following analytical phase.

4.4   Analytical Phase

In strategic debriefing, the questions posed by the debriefer become the tool to induce the learner to feel things differently and therefore to change his reactions, helping him to discover his own resources that were previously blocked by previous perceptions, sometimes rigid and pathogenic.

The questions are initially open-ended, more general, and broader and then undergo a spiral process that, depending on the participant's answers, become structured around the particular characteristics of the situation, highlighting critical points.

For example, at the beginning of the conversation, you could highlight key elements through self-assessment, using the "plus/delta" method, in which the facilitator asks open-ended questions like "What went well?", "What is the best thing you did?" (plus) and "What could be changed?", or "What would you do differently?" (delta).

Alternatively, or in a complementary way, the debriefer can start with questions that begin with "Who, Where, How, When, What" and will be open-ended, i.e., questions that do not contain the answer in themselves and therefore do not create prejudice and a fear of being judged in the learner and at the same time allow the debriefer to orient himself.

However, using only open-ended questions and/or the plus/delta method runs the risk of not changing participants' attitudes but only proposing superficial reflections regarding the scenario performed. For this reason, it is good that this type of conversation is considered a bridge to methods, such as the strategic dialogue we propose, which not only deepen the causes of the observed results but also promote the change of participants' attitudes.

For example, in a *leadership* debriefing, the first question asked of the group might be "Was there a *leader*?", and then "Who?" The first is a typical open-ended question that does not imply any answer (otherwise it would be asking "who was the *leader*?": in this case, the question implicitly acknowledges that there was a *leader* anyway). The second question begins to tighten the circle, asking the group to comment on who led the team. Having defined the *leadership* hypothesis, the next question is asked of the "presumed *leader*": "Did you feel like a *leader*?" With this question, we explore the student's feeling, preparing him to reflect on his actions. After his eventual confirmation, we go deeper by asking the motivations for his feeling, that is, from what behaviors, verbal and nonverbal, has he understood that he was/is the leader. In essence: "What did you do to be a *leader*?" A *leader can* be recognized by the way he acts toward the group, and this should be brought out by the *leader* himself and immediately afterward confirmed by asking the same question to his collaborators: "Why did you feel he was a *leader*? Which of his behaviors led you to this conclusion?"

After exploring the de facto *leader*, the debriefer will turn to the group to find confirmation of *leadership* recognition. This agreement acts as positive reinforcement for the *leader* and for the group itself. At this point and only when the learner has become aware of his or her experience through the open-ended questions can the debriefer reinforce the agreement with a series of closed-ended questions with an illusion of alternatives, which are structured questions with only two possible answers.

These kinds of questions are not simply instruments of knowledge, but instruments of intervention in the direction of change, as they provoke in the learner new ways of feeling and reacting to his reality that were previously trapped in his perceptions, sometimes dysfunctional [3]. A typical question to the illusion of alternative could be: "so do you think the *leader* should concentrate on doing the therapy, perhaps losing sight of the big picture, or remain outside the group action, to better coordinate the group itself?" In this case, the learner, having already recognized that it is better for the *leader* to remain outside the group to better coordinate, through this further question to the illusion of alternative, receives a further perceptive reinforcement of the correctness of his discovery made during the scenario by the debriefer.

At this point, before proceeding further, the debriefer will use the tool of paraphrasing [3] that confirms that the reflection is going in the right direction and that allows for the anchoring of the perception of the learner to the new perspective with respect to the experience of the scenario.

For example: "Correct me if I am wrong, NN organized and coordinated the work, stopped the group every now and then with a 10 × 10 re-evaluation of the clinical situation, did not take an active part in the practical activities and was able to listen to his team. I would say that these are all typical actions of a *leader*." By saying "correct me if I'm wrong," you make the learners feel that they are the ones leading the process of the discovery dialogue. In this way, they will not feel disqualified, but rather gratified. This restitution by the debriefer of the learners' discoveries in the form of paraphrases also serves to reinforce the discoveries, highlighting how they came about from below and not imposed a priori by the debriefer, who in turn reaffirms, in this way, his role as "facilitator" and not "teacher."

"The same words in different sequences produce different results." This statement by Pascal fits well with the methodology of the restructuring paraphrase. This is the maneuver that the debriefer performs each time he manages to define a problem with each of the participants after having asked open-ended questions and then, under the illusion of alternatives, obtains a redefinition of the problem that occurred during the scenario. No evaluation or interpretation is proposed, but with a modest "correct me if I'm wrong," "if I've understood correctly," and therefore non-judgmental attitude, the verification of the learning process and the understanding of the problem that was presented is asked, obtaining at the same time an openness to new perspectives and solutions proposed by the pupil himself and/or his teammates. Paraphrasing creates a climate of collaborative relationship between the debriefer and learner and circumvents possible misunderstandings and resistance. The learner feels accepted and is put in the first person, author of the discovery made about the problem presented and of its resolution.

In addition, it helps consolidate in the student the conviction that even if one has made mistakes, the most important thing is what one does with those mistakes because, as Huxley says, "reality is not what happens to us, but what we do with what happens to us."

After the first set of questions, we start to delve into the "funnel." Continuing the example of the *leadership* theme, it is good to delve into the specific aspects and how they were conducted during the scenario. The first deepening question, exploring the leader and his team, will be asked in a positive way, always starting from the general, "What was the best thing you did?" and "What was the best thing done by the leader?" and then going into detail: "What positive actions of the leader toward the patient (diagnosis, treatment, etc.) did you appreciate most?" "What were the *leader*'s most positive actions toward the team?" Starting with the positive actions, one can move down the funnel by exploring "what could have been done differently," that is, what could have been improved. You can explore, for example, workload distribution, closed-loop communication, awareness, listening skills, etc.

After a series of open-ended questions, possibly followed by the illusion of alternative questions, the debriefer can paraphrase again to get the group's agreement on what has been analyzed. If there is sufficient material, the debriefer can use a restructuring paraphrase associated with an evocative sentence. The technique always consists of using the learner's answers to reformulate the definition of the problem, but this time, rhetorical figures that fit the topic and the learner's feelings are used, to facilitate change, because "if you want to persuade someone, do it through his own arguments" (Aristotle). In the case of the debriefing on *leadership*, we could, as an example, summarize as follows: "we therefore saw that NN was a good *leader*; in fact, he took charge of the situation, delegated appropriately, asked his head teacher for advice, and accepted the proposals of his collaborators. However, he could have been more careful when the patient's condition suddenly changed. But thanks to the intervention of the anesthetist and the suggestions of the nurse who promptly flagged the monitor parameters, there were no problems. On the contrary, thanks to teamwork, the patient improved rapidly! Even a good conductor can sometimes be out of tune in some details, but if he conducts real masters, the orchestra can cover the out-of-tune." The feeling that we want to evoke is that the team is composed of professionals (the masters of the orchestra) and not of simple collaborators or gregarious professionals, who can represent a barrier to any errors or oversights of the *leader*.

Evocative language uses all kinds of rhetorical figures and poetic forms: aphorisms, metaphors, anecdotes, concrete examples, narratives, or counternarratives. This technique is used to create aversion toward attitudes or behaviors that need to be interrupted or changed or encouragement toward those reactions that need to be stimulated or increased.

According to the *Collins English Dictionary*, a metaphor is "an imaginative way of describing something by referring to something else which is the same in a particular way." The model, parable, fable, allegory, and myth are all subclasses of metaphor [9].

Metaphors are used by the debriefer to help participants in the scenario to see things differently and have different reactions. They are less threatening and provocative than direct statements and are a useful communication model to establish a good relationship with one's learners. According to Watzlawick and Nardone [6], metaphor is the language of the right cerebral hemisphere, the one that processes information simultaneously and holistically, and includes nonverbal language. It is the language that induces change.

For example, a nurse frustrated by the apparent futility of his or her marginal role during a highly complex specialty scenario might recognize (and discover) at the end of the strategic questions posed by the debriefer that his or her suggestions have resulted in improved therapeutic outcomes. The debriefer, instead of stopping to note the learner's discovery, might use persuasive language to reinforce, in a more performing manner, the positive attitude that could prove decisive in actual practice. For example, he might say, "Knowing how to propose can sometimes help someone (the *leader*) who is in a position where they can't see or hear. A good team member is sometimes the eye and ear of the *leader....*"

4.5 Application Phase

When the debriefer is aware that each of his or her learners has brought home a result, we move, as in standard debriefing, to the application phase. In this phase, each learner is asked to share what they have learned by carrying out the scenario, and during the debriefing, the typical question in this phase is, "What are you taking home?" Often, the learner stays on the surface and reports taking home a generic "I learned that it is important to communicate." Strategic debriefing introduced the concept, borrowed from strategic *problem-solving*, of goal setting [10]. In concrete terms, the student not only is asked to share what he has learnt but is also encouraged to reflect on how the debriefing experience can represent the first step toward a personal change that can, in turn, determine a positive change in the clinical activity in the hospital. To do this, the definition of a SMART goal is introduced [11]: (S) specific, i.e., concrete and clear; (M) measurable, i.e., defined in terms of observable results; (A) actionable, i.e., truly feasible; (R) achievable, based on constraints and resources; and (T) timed, i.e., achievable in a given period of time. The debriefer will then pose the question in such a way that the "I'm personally taking home" responds to the realization of a goal that is SMART, and, in particular, is the smallest actionable step, and dependent only on the learner, toward concrete change. The setting of a goal that is SMART by the learner is the result of a good strategic debriefing.

For example, usually, after a traditional debriefing to the question "What did you learn? What are you taking home with you?", the participant usually responds, "I've learned that it's important to communicate using the closed-loop method." After a strategic debriefing, the answer might instead be: "By next week, at the first emergency that happens to me, I will make my request to the nurse by calling him/her by name, looking him/her in the eyes and asking for feedback on the action taken."

At the end of the application phase, the debriefer can again use evocative language, quickly redefining the goal of change for each student (or for the whole group) and then using an "echo effect" closure that leaves a suggestion, using a short sentence (aphorism, story, anecdote, quotation) that functions as an anchor and emotional stabilization of the discovery made by the students.

4.6 General Considerations

Strategic communication allows debriefers greater effectiveness in both low- and high-fidelity simulations. The simulation method fits and complements strategic communication well. Both aim to bring about change, which must first be experienced and then explained.

The central fulcrum on which Watzlawick and Nardone's brief strategic therapy is based [5] is the corrective emotional experience in which the patient modifies his vision of reality through concrete emotional experiences. Similarly, those who participate in a strategic debriefing after a simulated scenario live a corrective emotional experience and are helped to break their perceptual patterns, triggering the premises for a real change in their clinical behavior that will persist over time.

In fact, in order for change to be rapid and effective, it must first produce a real experience of transformation at the perceptual-emotional level in the person, and only then can it be the subject of cognitive reasoning. In other words, the change must first pass through the experience and emotion phase and only then to the level of cognitive awareness; in fact "There is nothing in the intellect that has not first been in the senses" (St. Thomas Aquinas).

Strategic language, an effective tool in short-term strategic psychotherapy and in business *problem-solving*, is ideal and complementary to the simulation method, making it more performing and functional since, alongside common logic, it makes use of non-ordinary logical language.

4.7 Psychotraps and Their Use in Simulation

In this section, we will define and describe some of our mental attitudes (psychotraps) that are also recurrent in debriefing participants.

Knowledge of the main psychotraps and their possible solutions (psychosolutions) is an additional tool that can be used by the strategic debriefer during the simulation sessions.

As is well known, our mind in its psychophysiological processes responds to the need to reduce the expenditure of energy, and for this reason, it tends to work through schematizations and functional associations. This is why it elaborates the processes that have allowed us to solve certain problems and tends to transform them into replicable schemes when faced with similar situations. That is, we tend to always apply the same solution when it has always worked previously for that type of problem (generalization process). However, a situation can only be generalized for the class of problems for which it has been successfully formulated and applied.

In some cases, the similarity with similar situations deceptively leads us to the perception that they are the same circumstances or to think that what has worked for a similar problem will work, at least in part, with the solution that we usually find successful in that case. In essence, the human mind tends to repeat what has worked, but if the circumstances change, that solution is no longer functional or is not so automatically and so becomes a dysfunctional solution. The reiteration of a dysfunctional solution generates a psychotrap [12].

Even clinicians in their clinical behaviors often insist on applying what has been successful in the past, without keeping in mind that even the same problem in different circumstances may require different solutions. Simulation and strategic debriefing help participants identify clinical behaviors that hide dysfunctional psychotraps that may be at the root of medical errors.

Giorgio Nardone and his school of brief strategic therapy and strategic *coaching* and *problem-solving* have identified seven psychotraps of thinking and eight psychotraps of acting and their corresponding strategic solutions. We will examine those that occur most often during simulation and debriefing.

4.7.1   The Deception of Expectations

This psychotrapic trap is the most frequent. It consists of the tendency to attribute our perceptions and beliefs to others while expecting them to do the same as we do. We expect others to do what we would do in their place. This psychotrap is based on our inability to take on different points of view in evaluating reality, and its solution is to learn to observe reality through the eyes of others. An example is the "tunnel vision" that occurs with considerable frequency in medical emergencies, which consists of trying to solve a problem over and over again in the exact same way, without realizing it, even when it is clear that no result will be achieved.

There are three main types of fixation errors that result in "tunnel vision" [13]:

- "This and only this..." is the persistent fixation on a single problem, failing to review the diagnosis or plans, despite evidence that contradicts you. In some cases, the available evidence is interpreted out of the clinical context; in others, the secondary problems capture attention at the expense of the primary (e.g., treating the tachycardia instead of the major bleeding, etc.).

– "Anything but this...": it is the persistent inability to act on the main problem. Considerable time is wasted looking for other causes, sometimes to the exclusion of dealing with the main cause.

– "All is well...": it is the dogged belief that there is no major problem. Generally, some reassuring signs are overrated to override the more worrisome evidence (e.g., despite anuria and increased lactates, the patient is conscious, so no urgency to treat the patient, etc.). Similarly, worrisome data are deleted and considered artifactual, despite other concomitant data indicating impending deterioration.

Simulation, through the rules of CRM, suggests preventing this issue with "a view from above," taking on ever-changing perspectives. In high-fidelity simulation, a good exercise to avoid this psychotrapic trap is to practice role switching in scenarios. By playing a different role from the one usually experienced in real life, the learner becomes more aware of the ways of thinking and acting of a colleague or collaborator belonging to another discipline. In practice, the Heinz Von Foerster suggestion is made: "Always behave in such a way as to increase your possibilities of choice."

4.7.2 The Illusion of Ultimate Knowledge

Very often, we believe that we can achieve anything through knowledge and study. We believe that error in medicine can be prevented by greater attention, by scientific updating, or by implementing individual and organizational performance. It is a common belief that the expert, or the most senior in service, is always right, that more information equals more knowledge, that the most recent findings (e.g., the most recent therapy) are always the best, or that following guidelines protects us from errors and always guarantees success. However, with simulation, we learn that "knowing" or "knowing how to do" is almost always not enough but that perception and emotion can also significantly influence our behavior and clinical knowledge. In practice, we discover that the linear principle of cause and effect does not apply to most complex phenomena such as those that occur during a medical emergency.

The solution is to always maintain an unaltered skepticism without locking oneself up in reassuring certainties, learning to keep at bay the normal propensity to reassure ourselves through apparent scientific certainties that in reality are only consolatory self-deceptions, because "men see in matter an order that they have placed there" (Pascal).

4.7.3   The Myth of Perfect Reasoning

We have often been educated and trained with this psychotrap: through reasoning and rational logic, all problems can be solved. Hegel says: "If the theory does not agree with the facts, so much the worse for the facts." Especially during an emergency, it is not uncommon to ignore symptoms that do not agree with one's diagnostic hypothesis, to make fixation and tunnel errors, and to follow uncritically and blindly prescribed procedures. We are convinced that "if I use only logic while ignoring emotions and perceptions, my performance will be better." If we have to make a diagnostic-therapeutic decision, the use of rational logic will be of great help, but if we have to overcome an emotional impasse that may accompany us during our clinical practice, we must resort to different tools. Managing logic too rigidly can also become dysfunctional. By practicing the scenarios proposed by the simulation, we learn to see that linear logic, which we use daily with success in our clinical activity, can be a hindrance when we face emergencies with high emotional impact (for us and/or for our colleagues and our patients) and that we must therefore learn to manage and let flow even our (or their) most hidden and unrecognized emotions that can greatly interfere with the cognitive processes that are required to face the clinical situation.

4.7.4   I Felt It, Then Is

It is the psychotrapic that stands at the opposite end of the previous one (that of 4.7.3). As with all the psychotraps previously described, the fact applies that it is not the behavior itself but its rigid application to any problem that can turn a successful behavior into a dysfunctional one for that specific occasion. In this case, it is a matter of making decisions without any analytical rigor or clinical evidence. Trusting only one's clinical sense and intuition, perhaps just because that's how I've always gotten good results, could be the source and cause of medical error. Simulation helps teach us that "feeling" must coexist with "acting" so that they control each other.

4.7.5   Consistency at All Costs

One falls into this psychotrap when coherence, from a useful tool of logic, is transformed into a dogmatic procedure: it has always been done this way; this is what I was taught and what I have learned to do; I have made the right diagnosis, and it cannot be otherwise; I have made a diagnosis, and it cannot be changed in such a short time: "it is our theories that determine our observations" (Einstein). This happens when one is rigid and incapable of adapting in a flexible way to changes in clinical reality which, especially in emergencies, is rapidly changing. CRM suggests the use of the method of continuous reassessment as a solution, which must be constantly exercised by both the *leader* and the team during simulation scenarios.

4.7.6 Overestimate/Underestimate

At the base of this psychotrap is Festinger's theory of cognitive dissonance, according to which human beings, once they have made a decision, look for all the evidence that confirms it and avoid anything that proves its falsehood. The consequence is that we tend to overestimate or underestimate.

We use double standards for the same situation depending on the relationship we have with the subject at stake, and often that subject is us. It has been demonstrated that when our self-esteem and competence are at stake, the safety of our patient can be easily overlooked as we tend to protect ourselves. Thus, some reassuring signs may be overestimated in order to reassure ourselves, while more worrying signs may be underestimated or ignored for the same reason.

Simulation helps the learner discover that medical error is primarily a systems error (see Chap. 1) and that good teamwork can protect against the sometimes-inevitable individual fallacy.

References

1. Capogna, G., Capogna, E., & Nardone, G. (2020). The strategic debriefing. Incorporating strategic dialogue into the standard debriefing after the scenario. *MedEdPublish, 9*(1), 210.
2. Nardone, G., & Watzlawick, P. (1993). *The art of change: Strategic therapy and hypnotherapy without trance.* Jossey-Bass.
3. Nardone, G., & Salvini, A. (2004). *The strategic dialogue.* Ponte alle Grazie.
4. Watzlawick, P., Beavin, J. H., & Jackson, D. D. (1971). *Pragmatics of human communication.* Astrolabe.
5. Watzlawick, P., & Nardone, G. (1997a). *Brief strategic therapy.* Cortina.
6. Watzlawick, P., & Nardone, G. (1997b). *The language of change: Elements of therapeutic communication.* Feltrinelli.
7. Spering, M., Wagener, D., & Funke, J. (2005). The role of emotions in complex problem solving. *Cognition and Emotion, 19*, 1252–1261.
8. Nardone, G. (2019). *Emotions. Instructions for use.* Ponte alle Grazie.
9. Turbayne, C. M. (1970). *The myth of metaphor.* University of South Carolina Press.
10. Nardone, G., Mariotti, R., Milanese, R., Fiorenza, A. (2000). *La terapia dell'azienda malata.* Ponte alle Grazie.
11. Doran, G. T. (1981). There's a S.M.A.R.T. way to write management's goals and objectives. *Management Review, 70*(11), 35–36.
12. Nardone, G. (2013). *Psychotraps.* Ponte alle Grazie.
13. DeKeyser, V., & Woods, D. D. (1990). Fixation errors: Failures to revise situation assessment in dynamic and risky systems. In A. G. Colombo & A. S. Bustamante (Eds.), *Systems reliability assessment.* Kluwer.

Strategic Debriefing in Practice

5

Most people listen with the intention of responding, not with the desire to understand.

A.C. Doyle

The purpose of debriefing after the scenario is to reinforce the learning associated with a practical experience, i.e., to discuss in a structured way what happened during the scenario in the context of medical practice, considering both clinical and technical events and behavioral, non-technical events, and to extrapolate what has been learned to similar clinical situations.

How to identify and choose the objectives of the scenario was covered in Sect. 2.2.

In this chapter, we will describe, for each of the debriefing phases, a basic and an advanced strategic model (Table 5.1).

The basic template can be used as a guide for those who are starting out as facilitators or for those who have little experience but want to achieve a reliable and safe result quickly. It can also be used when you want to debrief exclusively on technical skills or when you are dealing with learners who are students or are particularly inexperienced.

Advanced strategic debriefing is the more advanced version, reserved for experienced facilitators who want to improve and further deepen their debriefing techniques, or for those finding themselves having to facilitate a group of colleagues who have had repeated experiences in simulation, or who are already competent in the subject but wish to especially deepen communication skills and strategies.

Advanced strategic debriefing is not an alternative debriefing, but should rather be considered as complementary, so the debriefer should start with one or more standard techniques and then continue, to deepen and make the educational message more efficient and persistent, using the strategic technique.

The debriefing model that will be described is based on the previously described and most commonly used models, supplemented and updated by the strategic dialogue techniques we have introduced.

G. Capogna et al., *Strategic Debriefing for Advanced Simulation*, https://doi.org/10.1007/978-3-031-06104-2_5

Table 5.1 Specific fields of application of strategic debriefing

	Standard Debriefing	Strategic Debriefing
Debriefer skills	Also beginner	Expert
Participant skills	Any	Preferably advanced
Skills explored	Techniques, Behavioral	Techniques, Behavioral, Emotional
Purpose	Improved performance as a result of logical-rational awareness	Change in performance resulting from a corrective emotional experience

5.1 Briefing Before the Scenario

In order to illustrate how the strategic approach performs better, even during the briefing, we describe a possible example of how the manikin and the simulation room can be presented (the environment where the scenario will take place and the equipment in it) in a strategic manner.

Usually, the manikin and the environments are presented for what they are: a dummy and a simulation room.

The debriefer or instructor usually begins the briefing preceding the scenario by explaining the manikin as follows: "For this scenario you will be using a state-of-the-art manikin that can simulate almost all human physiological functions including pregnancy. It is equipped with peripheral wrists and a heartbeat that can simulate any frequency and rhythm. It can be auscultated, and you will be able to hear both vesicular murmur and pathological lung sounds. The manikin is ventilatable and may be intubated; it can simulate any difficulty with the airway because it can also simulate difficult airways…It can deliver a baby, and it can bleed, and you will be able to insert a bladder catheter…etc. For the scenario, you will be asked to imagine that you are in the operating room or the delivery room or the emergency room or the ward. Now I will explain how to do therapy, how to draw blood samples, how to send them, and how to call for help…now try all the features I have outlined…do you have any questions?"

Basically, in this first version, the instructor provides more or less detailed instructions on how the manikin works and what its functional limits are (e.g., it cannot become edematous, it cannot gain weight, it cannot become cyanotic so you need to adjust with saturation, etc.), basically explaining what is real, what is realistic, and what you need to imagine is true during the scenario.

But there is also another way of presenting the high-fidelity manikin. In keeping with the general principles of simulation that "we learn by doing" and the principles of strategic dialogue that we empathize better if things are "felt inside" and not "instructed from the outside," the same explanation could be done in this other way:

The debriefer enters the simulation room with the participants and addresses the patient (the manikin) directly: "Good morning Madam, what is your name? How old are you? Could you please tell me about your first pregnancy? Let me introduce you to some colleagues…." Addressing the manikin and treating it exactly as if it was a patient immediately makes it clear to all participants that it is not about pretending. The "patient" responds, interacts with the learners who after a short time feel involved and begin to treat the manikin as if it was a real person, entering, almost without realizing it, into the "contract of realistic pretending" that is necessary for the scenario to run smoothly. "Do you mind if I show these colleagues how they can take your blood pressure? Could we try to listen to your heart?" Each feature is not explained but is performed and shared by and with the learners. "Is there anyone who has never put in a bladder catheter? Are there any nurses among you? Would you like to have your colleague experience how to put in a catheter?" This moment of training in the use of the manikin is a great opportunity for the debriefer to let his or her trainees experience shared circular learning: everyone can teach something to someone else. It will be easier in this way, when debriefing, to obtain a favorable atmosphere, open to mutual learning. The debriefer does not do, does not direct, but facilitates the process of harmoniously sharing the skills that each of the participants already possesses, adding what is needed to achieve the skills necessary to adequately perform the scenario. Often, when one has to try the maneuver of bladder catheterization, the patient, if not warned beforehand, can complain, drawing in a meta-communicative way the attention of the participants to the fact that one is in front of a real patient. The same technique is used to illustrate the environmental functionalities, one "is" in an operating room, and therefore one behaves as one usually does in an operating room and does not "pretend" that this is an operating room: in practice, the debriefer passes from explanations of the type "instructions for use" directly to "let's do as if" and acts and behaves himself as if he were in an operating room. Once the confidence of the participants has been built up, they can begin to point out differences with the real world, such as how to phone for advice, how to take a blood sample, or how to inject a drug for therapy. The more confident the participants become in the realism of the environment that the debriefer is presenting to them, the more they will notice the similarities with the real world and not the differences, maintaining that realism which is essential and functional to the good performance of the scenario itself.

5.2 What to Do During the Scenario

Usually a high-fidelity simulation scenario using full-scale manikins takes place within a simulation room, with an adjacent control room, equipped with cameras and glass panes that allow observation without being seen by participants. The debriefer in this case, after the briefing, will position himself inside the control room, together with the simulation technician and other members of the simulation center staff and any other co-debriefers.

Other types of simpler scenarios or in situ intra-hospital simulation situations may instead involve the presence of the debriefer within the simulation site.

In all cases, the debriefer has the task of observing and remembering the scenario, the behavior of each participant, and the critical issues that arose, noting the technical and behavioral skills used or lacking, in accordance with the objectives set, but being careful to identify all further learning opportunities offered by the scenario itself. Basically, in this observation phase, the debriefer should identify what will then be the topics that will be highlighted during the debriefing.

To make a good debriefing, it is therefore necessary to be a good and careful observer in the control room, but even the most experienced debriefer may have difficulty in identifying and remembering everything, so we suggest some techniques to use. First of all, it is not recommended for the inexperienced debriefer to have an active role in the scenario management in order to avoid a high cognitive load.

As a rule, unless you are really experienced, it is good to have the script in advance and not improvise a debriefing on a scenario you don't know.

Tools or checklists can be used to capture critical elements based on the training objectives and used during debriefing to conduct critical reflection and not forget anything.

For technical skills, the checklist of critical actions specific to that scenario can be used based on the training objectives of that scenario (e.g., performing primary ABCDE assessment, performing orotracheal intubation, etc.).

For non-technical skills, there are a number of models in the literature that indicate those behavioral markers deemed important to successful operational practices with maximum safety. An example of a scheme to follow for assessing non-technical skills is the Ottawa *Crisis Resource Management Global Rating Scale* (Fig. 5.1), which uses a 1–7 measurement scale with clear definitions of standards and identifies, five specific dimensions (*leadership*, problem-solving, situational awareness, resource utilization, and communication), and an overall *performance* [1, 2].

It is very useful to make a note of the time when you observe key actions that take place and that we think are important to discuss in the debriefing afterward. Some examples of practical cards for the debriefer in training are shown in Fig. 5.2: these cards can be used to fix critical issues and positive actions and to easily track down the right time should you then want to use video to draw the attention of learners during debriefing. A more sophisticated alternative are some video-capture systems supplied with the software that manages the manikin, which allow you to insert tags, with different colors according to the category of event (*communication*, *procedural abilities*, etc.), and to make annotations in order to quickly find the salient moments.

For more complex multidisciplinary high-fidelity scenarios, even the most experienced debriefer has never to worry about the technical running of the scenario (such as the voice of the patient-dummy, operating the functions of the dummy, answering the telephone, worrying about the materials, supervising the smooth

OVERALL PERFORMANCE

1	2	3	4	5	6	7
Novice; all CM skills require significant improvement		Advanced novice; many CM skills require moderate improvement		Competent; most CM skills require minor improvement		Clearly superior; few, if any CM skills that only require minor improvement

I. LEADERSHIP SKILLS

1	2	3	4	5	6	7
Loss calm and control for most of crisis; unable to make firm decisions; cannot maintain global perspective		Loss calm/control frequently during crisis; delays in making firm decisions (or with cueing); rarely maintain global perspective		Stay calm and in control for most of crisis; makes firm decisions with little delay; usually maintains global perspective		Remains calm and in control for entire crisis; makes prompt and firm decisions without delay; always maintains global perspective

II. PROBLEM SOLVING SKILLS

1	2	3	4	5	6	7
Cannot implement ABC's assessment without cues; uses sequential management despite cues; fails consider any alternative in crisis		Incomplete or slow ABC's assessment; mostly uses sequential management approach unless cued; gives little consideration to alternatives		Satisfactory ABC assessment without cues; mostly uses concurrent management approach with only minimal cueing; considers some alternative in crisis		Thorough yet quick ABC assessment without cues; always uses concurrent management approach; considers most likely alternative in crisis

III. SITUATION AWARNESS SKILLS

1	2	3	4	5	6	7
Becomes fixated easily despite repeated cues; fails reassess and re-evaluates situation despite repeated cues; fails to anticipated likely events		Avoids fixation error only with cues; rarely reassess and re-evaluates situation without cues; rarely anticipates likely events		usually avoids fixation error with minimal cueing; reassesses and re-evaluates situation frequently with minimal cues; usually anticipates likely events		Avoids fixation error only without cues; constantly reassesses and re-evaluates situation without cues; constantly anticipates likely events

III. RESOURCE UTILIZATION SKILLS

1	2	3	4	5	6	7
Unable to use resources and staff effectively; does not prioritize tasks or ask for help when required despite cues		Able to use resources and staff with minimal effectiveness; only prioritizes tasks or asks for help when required with cues		Able to use resources and staff with moderate effectiveness; able to prioritize tasks and/or asks for help when required with minimal cues		Clearly able to use resources and staff to maximal effectiveness; sets clear task priority and asks for help with no cues

I. COMUNICATION SKILLS

1	2	3	4	5	6	7
Does not communicate with staff; does not acknowledge staff communication, never uses directed verbal/non-verbal communication		Communicates occasionally with staff but unclear and vague; occasionally listens to but rarely interacts with staff; rarely uses directed verbal/non-verbal communication		Communicates with staff clearly and concisely most of time; listens to staff feedback; usually uses directed verbal/non-verbal communication		Communicates clearly and concisely with staff at all time encourages input and listens to staff feedback; constantly uses directed verbal/non-verbal communication

Fig. 5.1 The Ottawa GRS [1]

running of the programs, etc.), which should therefore always be left to a qualified technician or another debriefer-colleague. The debriefer should be limited to purely observing the scenario unfolding, giving the technician, if and when necessary, any

Participant's name Role in the scenario Time	Participant's name Role in the scenario Time
Participant's name Role in the scenario Time	Participant's name Role in the scenario Time

Example A

Example B

Plus What did we do well?	Video (Min)	Delta Areas of improvements

Fig. 5.2 Examples of observation sheets for debriefers

elements for the development of the reactions of the manikin and the scenario in response to the participants' behavior.

The number and type of staff needed in the control room depend on the characteristics and complexity of the scenario, as well as the type of participants.

For example, in highly complex multidisciplinary scenarios, the following professionals would be needed in the control room:

- The debriefer who will be in charge of the participants' group from the briefing and who will lead the debriefing after the scenario
- The simulation technician, expert in the clinical development of the scenario and in the reactions of the manikin to the participants' behaviors, also responsible for the preparation of the scenario and of the materials connected to it
- A staff member, experienced in the scenario, who acts as the voice of the patient
- An auxiliary debriefer, who takes note of the timeline of the scenario, linking the time of the event reported by the debriefer with the video recording that can be used during the debriefing
- A staff member, familiar with the scenario, assigned to answer the phone, ready to enter the scene as an actor, and prepared for other auxiliary and support functions

If the debriefing is conducted by a debriefer and a co-debriefer, the "scopes of observation" can be divided by expertise, so that one debriefer may focus primarily on the technical component of the scenario (often being the content expert) and the other on the non-technical component.

5.3   Reaction and *De-roling* Phase

The phase immediately following the scenario and immediately preceding the debriefing after the scenario is the delicate phase of "exiting the role" or "reaction phase" or "defusing."

The purpose of this phase, usually of short duration (2–5 min), is to give participants time to deal with reactions and emotions, in order to get out of the role they had during the scenario, allowing them to participate in the debriefing with a lower emotional load. Typically, this phase takes place immediately after the end of the scenario, immediately before moving toward the debriefing room, but outside the simulation room where the scenario took place. It is important to capture the immediate, "hot" feelings of the learners in order to gain an understanding of their emotional state even if only by talking on the way from the simulation room to the debriefing room. Immediately upon leaving the scenario, animated conversation among participants is common, reflecting a normal emotional release. At the opposite end of the spectrum, an embarrassed silence may indicate a general perception that the simulated case was not handled well or that the case was not challenging enough. The debriefer must be skilled enough not to leave this time between the end of the scenario and the beginning of the debriefing to casual comments from the learners, but to be able to manage it by conducting a good *de-roling* quickly but effectively.

At this stage, participants need to realize that they have participated in a role play, albeit an unusual one, in the sense that they have played themselves. In fact, there may have been a conflict between what is real and what is not, and the scenario may have distorted the way participants have interpreted themselves and the role assigned. This can produce a strange emotional reaction of difficulty in identifying the boundaries between "the self" and "the act." So, it is important to recognize early on that there are reasons why the way they behaved in the scenario may not reflect the way they might behave in real life (e.g., dealing with simulated patient, lack of some clinical cues, awareness of being videotaped, uncertainty or confusion about some technical aspects of how to behave during a simulation, etc.).

If participants adopt a defensive position triggered by something that occurred during the scenario, it is necessary to address it briefly in order to reach an agreement (e.g., accept the limitation of the realism of the simulation, explain why the scenario was stopped, solve a misunderstanding, etc.) so that the reaction phase can proceed normally or, better, it can be postponed to a later elaboration during or after the debriefing, if you do not want to interrupt the flow of the participants' emotions. In the case of positive appreciation from the participants, one can already start to reinforce the idea that they have just had a unique opportunity to "learn in safety," by doing something that normally cannot be done, i.e., seeing themselves in action while interacting with a simulated clinical situation that is so realistic as to allow a precious and unrepeatable educational reflection.

If *de-roling is* not done properly, participants may be hampered in their ability to make the most of the debriefing session. This is somewhat comparable to what happens to those actors "stuck in the role," who get stuck with the feelings and emotions of their character that do not belong to them.

The logic behind this emotional phase of reaction is that an analysis of what has happened cannot be done correctly by the left hemisphere of the brain while the right hemisphere is still "occupied" by a flow of emotions.

5.3.1 In Basic Debriefing

In a basic debriefing, the typical question that the debriefer asks the participants in this phase is "How do you feel?" or "How did you feel during the scenario?", and the answer that one wants to obtain from the trainees, or better, from every single trainee, is the description of the sensation evoked.

The question should be asked to each of the participants, and, in theory, it would be good to ask the question first to the youngest participant to avoid the "hierarchy effect" (the youngest could answer as the oldest has already answered) or, alternatively, to the participant who seems the most available. It is important to reiterate that the question is related to the feeling and emotion aroused by the scenario and not to the behaviors or contents of the scenario that will be discussed later, during the debriefing.

So, all comments, questions, and any discussions about how it went, what I could have done, what happened, etc. should be deferred and participants invited to resubmit their questions and comments during the debriefing.

By focusing the question on "how do you feel?", the learner is able to vent his emotion by telling his feelings, and the debriefer can investigate the participants' moods evoked by the scenario that could condition or explain the following dialogue during the debriefing.

5.3.2 In Strategic Debriefing

As usual, this phase must take place immediately after the end of the scenario and outside the simulation area, just before moving toward the debriefing room. This timing is crucial because the act of removing the surgical gowns as soon as they leave the simulation room is a ritual [3] and physical metaphor of their de-roling. Making the ritual of taking off the uniform coinciding with the moment of verbalizing one's emotions helps to step out of the role and to better manage the emotions felt. They then move immediately into the debriefing phase.

In case the debriefer wants to use strategic dialogue, this can certainly help him/her better highlight the emotions perceived by the participants immediately after the scenario.

In this case, the exploration of feelings and emotions is done in a more structured way with questions such as "In a very concise way, I would like to get an immediate impression of your emotions: What are you feeling right now? Does this feeling resonate with you in any way? Are there situations in your professional life or in your daily life that trigger this same feeling? Which ones? Is it the same or different from the previous scenario? If different, how?" The debriefer will afterward immediately use the technique of paraphrasing (see below) to summarize synthetically (e.g., "correct me if I'm wrong, you told me that you feel xxx and that this same feeling you usually experience in xy situations…") and will conclude with the next question, "Which of the four basic emotions, fear, pleasure, anger, and pain, do you relate this feeling to?", or, alternatively, hypothesize and propose to the learner the basic emotion that has pervaded him during or immediately after the scenario, asking for confirmation.

The learner may, for example, relate to the basic emotion of fear, his fear of making a mistake, or of being judged, or of not remembering the guidelines sufficiently; may relate to anger the feeling of not having performed a task that in real life is usually easy, or to his inability to communicate adequately; may relate to pleasure the feeling of a well performed team work and an effective and fluent communication with colleagues; and may relate to pain the memory of a previous unpleasant clinical event really experienced in the past, just evoked by the scenario.

In this way, the learner acquires the inner awareness of the real basic feeling/emotion that the scenario has aroused: evoking it, recognizing it, and becoming aware of it, he/she can let it flow, go along with the flow, and, with the help of the strategic debriefer, use it constructively. He will also be able to leave the role assigned to him in the scenario better and faster, making himself more willing to face the debriefing and to consider it as a personal cognitive learning tool, in which the performance (and not the person) and the environmental conditions that determined it are examined, in order to improve it in the future.

The debriefer will take note of the deep emotions that accompanied the participants during the scenario and can use them to better investigate the deep motivations for the behaviors during the subsequent debriefing phase.

Awareness of emotions is a cornerstone of change. Becoming aware of emotional experience and being able to verbalize it provide access to the adaptive information and action tendency inherent in each emotion. Once a person gets in touch with their "feeling," they can more easily connect to their needs (in this case learning needs) and motivate themselves to meet them (Speech Box 5.1).

"All our cognition begins in feelings" (Leonardo da Vinci): a good reaction phase paves the way for a good debriefing.

Speech Box 5.1 Typical Questions of the Reaction Phase

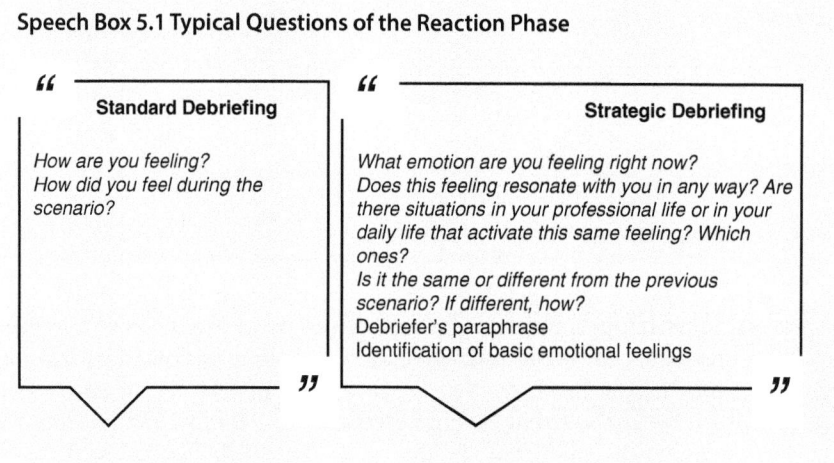

Standard Debriefing

How are you feeling?
How did you feel during the scenario?

Strategic Debriefing

What emotion are you feeling right now?
Does this feeling resonate with you in any way? Are there situations in your professional life or in your daily life that activate this same feeling? Which ones?
Is it the same or different from the previous scenario? If different, how?
Debriefer's paraphrase
Identification of basic emotional feelings

5.4   How to Start Debriefing: The Introduction to the Method

Before beginning the debriefing, it is necessary to have a plan and to establish an atmosphere conducive to learning. The established learning objectives should not necessarily be considered as the only key objectives of the debriefing, especially if other performance deficiencies have been observed leading to critical errors during the scenario. Flexibility and listening skills are two indispensable skills for conducting a good debriefing.

The debriefing is conducted in a different room from the one where the scenario took place, sitting in a circle or semicircle (if videotaping is to be used), with the debriefer sitting among the participants, to signify that the learning process in simulation is circular, non-unidirectional, non-judgmental, and "on an equal footing," i.e., that everyone can contribute to the learning of the other. The welcoming behavior of the debriefer as he seats each participant in the classroom is the first nonverbal sign that confirms the above.

The first thing to do is to thank the learners for their active participation in the simulation. This is a real and objective recognition of the fact that everyone has attempted to throw themselves fully into the scenario in order to learn and improve their clinical practice.

Immediately afterward, the debriefer must clearly state what the purpose of the debriefing is, "This is about improving one's own and the group's performance, not about criticizing anyone," and remind the trainees of the rules of the session, as they may be anxious to know how the debriefing will be conducted. Absence of judgment and confidentiality are two safety guarantees that need to be reiterated even if they were mentioned at the beginning of the course. For example, "There will be no judgment, criticism, or blame. Nothing discussed here will leave this room. We will speak one at a time without overlapping: what each of us says is too important not to deserve our full attention and listening; everyone learns from the other." Finally, it is important to inform participants about the structure of the debriefing itself, as they may not know what it is and how long it lasts. "There will be three different phases. The first, descriptive, in which we will describe what you saw and what happened; the second, analytical, in which we will analyze and try to understand what happened from different perspectives; and a third phase, or application phase, in which we will share what we learned from the scenario." The subdivision of the debriefing into phases has not only an informative intent but also, at a meta-communicative level, the purpose of presenting the debriefing as a working tool that as such can and must be learned and used by the learners.

Finally, if the scenario was stopped at a time that did not seem a natural or expected concluding step, the debriefer should give the reason, which is generally related to the learning objectives addressed. This will avoid participants starting the debriefing by describing what they were going to do next or complaining that it was unrealistic not to give them more time to complete the scenario.

5.5   Descriptive Phase

The descriptive phase aims to check each participant's understanding of what happened in the clinical case scenario. This serves both the participants, who clarify and briefly review the case and can begin to realize how their teammates experienced it, and the debriefer who begins to realize the experience of each of the participants.

5.5.1   In Basic Debriefing

Basically, in this phase, you explore what happened during the scenario through the eyes and narrative of the participants.

The description process consists of leading the group through an "agreed description" of the scenario that has just ended. This should be done on an action-by-action basis, limiting the discussion to the statement of facts and avoiding emotions and comments. The typical question in this phase is "What did you see?" or "What happened?" The focus should remain on creating a shared understanding of what actually happened in the scenario. Should any participant already want to enter into discussion or examine what went wrong or express any doubts, they should be gently stopped and invited to answer the question "what did you see?", reassuring them that all other points will be examined together shortly, in the next phase, and that for now it is important to reconstruct the course of the scenario.

If the learners have all entered the scenario together, you can ask the team leader to narrate what happened and then have the team complete the narrative.

If the learners have entered the scenario at different times, the question can be asked starting with the first to enter and then, in chronological order, to all the others. The advantage of this way of proceeding is that everyone can complete the other's story and/or become aware that if effective communication is not practiced, those who intervene when the scenario has already begun may have a very different view of the facts from those who entered first and vice versa.

The story of the scenario is thus recomposed through what everyone has seen and perceived and therefore experienced. This process is highly educational as it makes the participants realize, still in a subliminal way, that what they have experienced does not always coincide with the point of view of the other team member or *leader* and that there may be borderline cases in which no one or only a few had a clear idea of what it was about.

At the end of the round, the debriefer can turn to the *leader,* or more generically to everyone, and ask in a friendly way with an open-ended question: "So what was this scenario about?" If the answer is correct, the descriptive phase can be considered concluded; if there is no agreement, the discussion and analysis of the reasons for the lack of agreement or understanding by the participants (or some of them) is postponed to the analytical phase, which is the following one.

5.5.2   In Strategic Debriefing

In the case of advanced strategic debriefing, at the end of the descriptive phase, performed as described above, in accordance with the strategic dialogue, the debriefer uses the technique of paraphrasing (summarize to redefine) to summarize what happened as the participants experienced it.

For example: "If I understand correctly, correct me if I'm wrong, it was clear to everyone that this was a seizure that was identified early by the emergency room physician, who immediately called for help and together with his anesthesiologist colleague shared the decision-making process. The team was quickly able to stabilize the patient appropriately, even though it was unclear to the nurse what was causing the seizure. Did I get this right? Does anyone want to add anything further?" By synthetically reformulating the participants' experiences, the debriefer, in this way, establishes the starting point for the analytical phase and agrees with everyone's experiences, giving the trainees (and himself) the possibility to acquire a first awareness of possible performance deficiencies both in communicative and diagnostic-technical-therapeutic terms.

Moreover, in this way, the debriefer can also begin to define how much the experience and perceptions of each participant might have conditioned the behaviors during the scenario that will be discussed in the next analytical phase. Note how the debriefer never anticipates or suggests "the right answer," i.e., the diagnosis of the clinical case, but allows this to come out spontaneously from the learners. Only if this does not emerge from any of them will he clarify it in the final moment of the synthesis, which precedes the passage to the analytical phase.

The descriptive phase should last no longer than 10 min, or one quarter of the total debriefing duration (Speech Box 5.2).

Speech Box 5.2 Typical Questions of the Descriptive Phase

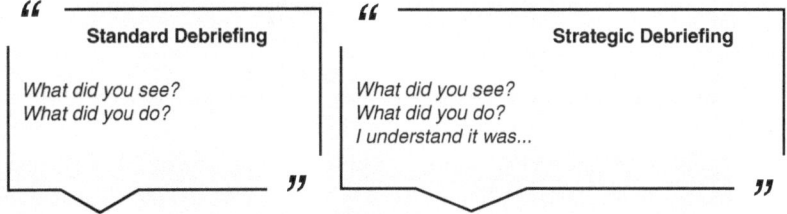

Standard Debriefing

What did you see?
What did you do?

Strategic Debriefing

What did you see?
What did you do?
I understand it was...

5.6   The Analytical Phase

The analytical phase (from the Greek *anàlisis* which means resolution) is the phase of deepening.

The general rules for the debriefer are:

1. The use of open questions, i.e., questions that do not contain, even implicitly, the answer. These are those that begin with "What, How, Why, and When."
2. A Socratic approach, in which the debriefer does not give information or direct answers to the participants' questions but is instead concerned with discovering the learners' answers, asking a series of questions so that the learners themselves arrive at the answer on their own or develop a deeper awareness of the limits of their knowledge.
3. The use of rephrasing a participant's question to himself and/or others, rather than giving direct answers too soon.
4. The use of active silence, understood as interested listening. If the debriefer does not speak, there will be someone who will take the floor.

5. Make it clear that it is not important who did the right things, but what is right for the patient. Criticism must be constructive: you can criticize the performance but not the person.
6. Special attention to body language.

In addition, the debriefer: (a) always has a plan (but not a rigid one); (b) involves each of the participants, restraining the more exuberant and facilitating the more timid; (c) highlights any key clinical and behavioral points not already highlighted by the participants; (d) points out that inappropriate actions taken during the scenario do not necessarily imply that they would have happened in the clinical setting, but one must question why they happened in the scenario, under those specific environmental conditions.

On the contrary, things to absolutely avoid are:

1. Have a debriefer-centered discussion (teaching and not facilitating, giving the impression that only one's opinion is the important one)
2. Give their opinion before the learners have said theirs
3. Interrupting participants or not listening carefully
4. Closed questions or questions that already contain the answer
5. Too rigid a set plan and not to identify or ignore learning opportunities offered by participants with their observations

Commonly, simulation centers are equipped with an audio-video system that allows live *streaming* and recording of scenarios. Theoretically, the video can be (a) entirely reviewed together with the participants before the beginning of the debriefing, (b) played and stopped every time there is something worth discussing, or (c) proposed by the debriefer during the analytical phase only if necessary and in short sequences concerning aspects to be deepened, or to point out to the participants some behaviors of which they were not aware. This third modality is the more commonly used and the one we consider the most appropriate. The video should be presented in a neutral tone and possibly associated with questions to collect participants' reactions. The same general rules of debriefing also apply to the video, so the sequences should not be used in a judgmental way, so phrases like "Look what you did wrong here!" are definitely to be proscribed. In most cases and if the clip has been well chosen, no comment is needed from the debriefer who can remain quietly silent as the video itself will speak for him/her. The video is a powerful but complementary tool and can be used by the debriefer when he wants to make observations or give suggestions without intervening directly. In this case, he can show some sequences so that the participants recognize and verify what happened, arriving at the answer by themselves, and this makes the learning more solid and stable because it is discovered by the individual and not suggested by others.

Each video sequence should be briefly introduced and contextualized by the debriefer, such as "Let's review this short film together now. It is about the moment when the analysis came in. What do you notice?"

5.6.1 In Basic Debriefing

For a "beginner" debriefer, the main problem is often how to begin the analytical phase.

A good method, simple but effective, is to start with a plus/delta approach [4] and then deepen with a series of open questions (why?) in a circular way, i.e., addressed to the person concerned, but then referred to the group and then back to the person concerned.

Typical questions in the plus/delta process basically summarize two concepts: what went well (plus) and what went wrong and could have been done better (delta) during the scenario.

There are many ways to ask these two questions.

The debriefer might ask participants, "What was successful about this simulation?", referring to the perceived results of the team, or "What was successful?" rather than "What do you think was successful?" which might imply that there was nothing good about it, or "What was good?", although this question might raise a moral issue between "good" and "bad," or even "What were the positive elements?", which might rightly make participants think that there are also negative elements on which they will be "judged" later. It is clear from these examples that the way the question is phrased can influence the answer and/or create a feeling among participants that hinders all learning efforts. In fact, it is quite different to ask "What did you do well?" or "Was there anything you did well?" which could also imply that maybe you didn't do anything, than asking "What was the best thing you did?" which lets the learner understand that they did many good things and that they are being asked to choose the best one. This is one of the most effective formulations of the first question in the plus/delta technique. It is in fact very powerful. Starting with the positives and, by so doing indicating that there have been positives, inviting the learner to report the best, usually pleasantly surprises the learner as they are usually mainly focused on seeing what went wrong or what they think they did wrong and expect criticism rather than praise. This first question sets him up well for the analytical process of debriefing. Moreover, it makes him discover how there are always positives, even unconscious, in our clinical behaviors. And if he cannot discover it by himself, the others in the team will help him. In fact, if, as sometimes happens, the learner does not find any positive aspect, the debriefer will have to ask the same question to the other members of the team, and usually there is always someone who has noticed positive attitudes in someone else. If the group can't find any positive behavior either, the debriefer, before reporting what he/she has noticed, can resort to an explanatory video sequence, which will give the answer that will certainly be much more powerful and effective than any statement he/she would make.

Obviously, the plus phase should be extended to each participant and, if desired, can be deepened to more than one aspect, depending on the progress of the debriefing and the time available.

The second part of the plus/delta technique focuses on the critical issues, i.e., the mistakes made, or, rather, the aspects to be improved (delta).

In fact, during a good debriefing, the question "What mistake did you make, what did you do wrong?" is never used and is replaced by "What could you have done better?", "What were the critical issues?", and "What could have been done differently?" One should never directly or indirectly accuse a learner of making a mistake as it violates the basic principles of psychological safety by contributing to raising defensive mechanisms that hinder any learning process.

Aspects for improvement are then explored with non-judgmental questions that can put participants at ease, such as "If you had to go back and redo the scenario, what would you do differently?" These types of questions should be asked of each of the participants who, with their answers, will elicit further exploration by the debriefer.

At this point, the debriefer can move on to explore in detail the reasons for the actions of the scenario participants by exploring the invisible mental frameworks behind the observed actions and their outcomes. The hypothesis is that there may have been erroneous mental frameworks or subjective perceptions that led to the wrong action(s) and that not knowing them could lead to a recurrence of bad decisions in the future. The typical insight question that helps investigate the basis and motivation for behaviors is "Why?" In this way, participants experience a very interactive debriefing that forces them to answer and reflect on what they did and what happened.

In an analysis that tends to delve into the deeper motivations for behaviors, the question containing the "why" may follow the more open-ended first question, such as the sequence:

What went well? Why did it go well?
What was difficult? Why was it hard?
What would you do next time? Why would you do that?

The circularity of questions is a very important aspect. The same question asked to one of the team members can be repeated to the others: "What do you think? Do you agree with it? Did you notice it too?" Confirmation by the group is an essential motivational element for those who are becoming aware of their behaviors during the scenario and how they could be improved (Speech Box 5.3).

Speech Box 5.3 Example of the Analytical Phase Sequence in the Basic Debriefing

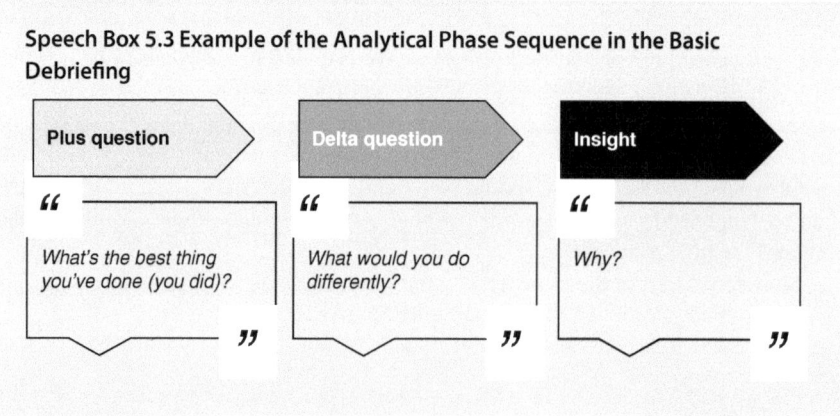

Plus question	Delta question	Insight
"	"	"
What's the best thing you've done (you did)?	What would you do differently?	Why?

Another way to start the debriefing is to directly ask an open-ended question regarding an observation made by the debriefer on a behavior that showed evident criticalities and/or that represented one of the previously established goals of the scenario. For example, in front of a confused scenario, where there was no mutual awareness of the team's actions and with difficulties in communication between the participants, the debriefer's first question could be: "How does communication seem to have gone?" Similarly, in a scenario with a lack of *leadership*, the first question might be, "Was there a *leader*?" If, on the other hand, the main purpose of the scenario was to practice technical guidelines, let's say on the difficult airway, and the participants had difficulty performing in practice, the first question would be, "How did you do with airway control?" Note that the questions are open-ended and do not assume judgment on the part of the debriefer, nor do they contain any commentary on the correctness of the execution of the procedures, leaving the participants free to express themselves without conditioning from the debriefer. This is followed by a series of open-ended questions, partly elicited by the participants themselves, which will be used by the debriefer to deepen the analytical phase. Speech Box 5.4 shows, as an example, a sequence of open questions. In general, when asking questions, the debriefer will look at the person to whom he/she wants to ask the question and call him/her by name so that it is clear to whom the question is directed. Asking questions in a general way to everyone is the same as asking no one at all, and you risk embarrassing silences, the response of the most exuberant, or the exclusion of the shyest.

Speech Box 5.4 Examples of Open Questions

"

Open Questions

What happened to this patient?
What was successful?
What difficulties did you encounter?
Overall, how did you feel you performed as a team?
What went right?
What has caused you frustration or embarrassment?
What surprised you about what you did?
How did you make your decisions?
How did you feel when it happened?
How did you understand that instruction?
What was happening at that moment?
What did you learn?
What/how would you do differently next time?
Why did you say this or that?
What do you think could be improved?
What else happened that caused the problem?

"

The classic form of in-depth inquiry that uses questions starting with "why?" to investigate the learners' mental framework is usually done when the learners are not beginners. Asking "Why?" directly might be difficult for beginners, such as young learners, because they may not yet possess a built mental framework or sufficient experience. Then the follow-up question might be along the lines of "What were you trying to do?"

A viable alternative with this type of participant is to use the technique of good judgment debriefing (*advocacy-inquiry*) [6, 7] which, as reported in Sect. 2.7.3, is a three-sentence process in which the first is the debriefer's neutral observation, "I observed that the patient assessment was delayed...."; the second is the reference to the debriefer's own mental picture, "I am concerned about this because for me it means that..."; and the third is the question called "of inquiry," "I would just like to know why the first action was to look at the patient's monitor settings...?" or "I wonder what I was thinking at the time."

In this case, instead of using a maieutic-type process in which he does not intervene directly but helps the learners to find the answers themselves, the debriefer first exposes what he noticed, precisely because of the learners' inexperience.

Note how the type of questions do not contain the direct "you" and that, although they are always addressed in a soft, non-judgmental way, they force one to answer and reflect on what one has done and what has happened. By avoiding the use of "you," the debriefer always refers to his own mental framework using "I." This type of approach promotes learning without offending the participants in any way and is extremely effective in exploring the reasons for critical or poor performance and their causes. Particular attention should be paid to the importance of the second sentence ("I'm concerned..."). If inadvertently the debriefer forgets this second sentence and moves from "I noticed this and this..." directly to "I just want to know why...", this may cause the young learner to feel accused or judged.

Whichever technique is used, in all cases, once the learner has identified his or her performance deficiency, this should be, so to speak, "closed" by the debriefer, and not left unresolved. In order to close it, three steps have to be followed: the first step (recapitulation) is the one in which the debriefer briefly summarizes the episode containing the error or criticality, asking the person concerned for confirmation. The second phase (generalization) is the one in which the rest of the group of participants is invited to enter into the matter with a sentence such as "Is there anyone who has had a similar experience during a similar situation or intervention?" In this way, the episode is decontextualized, and the impression is given to the participants that what happened can happen to everyone and is therefore of common interest. The third step (recontextualization) is to ask the learner himself for the solution to the problem, as this represents a much more powerful feedback than when the debriefer himself offers it. If the learner does not have any solution in mind, the debriefer proceeds to ask each of the other team members, such as "Do you know any strategies to solve a problem like this in the future?" Only if no one has a correct solution will the debriefer then suggest it.

At the end of these three steps, you can check again if the learner's learning was successful by asking him/her, "If you were to repeat the scenario, what would you do differently?" Or, "If a similar case were to happen to you in the hospital tomorrow, what would you do differently?"

When the debriefer is reasonably sure that each of his trainees has achieved a result, i.e., has reflected constructively on even a single technical or behavioral aspect, he can close the analytical phase and move on to the following application phase.

As with stories for which "there must be a length but one that is easy to embrace with memory" (Aristotle) so also for debriefing. It is more effective for learners to take home (learn) the didactic narrative they have produced rather than all the possible imaginable cues for discussion, perhaps superficially examined and only listed, but not deeply internalized.

The analytical phase should last, on average, no more than 30 min.

5.6.2   In Strategic Debriefing

In strategic debriefing, the questions, instead of simply guiding the debriefer and the participant to an understanding of the problem to be solved or the error committed, become the vehicle to induce the participant to feel things differently and therefore to change his reactions, helping him to discover his own resources that were blocked by previous perceptions, sometimes rigid and dysfunctional.

As in traditional debriefing, the questions are initially open-ended and then spiral around the learner's answers. As in standard basic debriefing, the debriefer can start with a plus/delta approach followed by open-ended questions (why?) or by directly asking an open-ended question regarding an observation made by the debriefer on a behavior that showed evident criticalities and/or that represented one of the predetermined objectives of the scenario.

When, and only after, the individual learner has discovered "on his own," through the debriefer's open questions and comparison with other participants, the causes of the technical-behavioral shortcomings of his actions during the scenario can the debriefer reinforce the discovery by using the technique of alternative illusion questions. These are closed questions, structured with only two possibilities of response. The debriefer can then choose which of the two best fits his case. Questions of this type are not only tools of knowledge but also of intervention in the direction of change, as they provoke in the learner new ways of feeling and reacting to his reality that were previously trapped in his perceptions. A typical alternative illusion question might be: "So do you think the *leader* should be doing practical things and losing sight of the big picture, or should he or she be outside the group action, to better coordinate the group?" In this case the learner, having already recognized that it is better for the *leader to be* outside the group to better coordinate, through this further alternative illusion question, receives further perceptive reinforcement of the correctness of his or her discovery made during the session by the debriefer. After hearing the favorable opinion of the rest of the group, which can also be externalized with a simple nonverbal behavior of assent, the debriefer, before proceeding further, will use the instrument of paraphrase [8] that confirms that the reflection is going in the right direction and that allows the trainees' perception to be anchored to the new perspective of the experience of the scenario. The paraphrase is the maneuver that the debriefer performs every time he/she manages to define a problem with each of the learners after having asked open-ended questions and then under the illusion of alternatives, obtaining the redefinition of the problem occurred during the scenario. In the paraphrase, no evaluation or interpretation is proposed but a verification of the process of learning and understanding of what has been presented is asked, encouraging an openness to new perspectives and solutions proposed by the participants themselves. For example, after a series of open and then closed confirmation questions, the learner who had the role of *leader* understands that he was able to communicate efficiently with the team but realized, watching the video recording of the scenario, that when the patient got worse, he started to measure the pressure, leaving the rest of the team waiting for dispositions. The debriefer could confirm his student's discovery by, for example, paraphrasing as follows: "If I understand correctly, correct me if I'm wrong, the *leader* distributed the workloads fairly and managed to converse with his team effectively, but when the patient suddenly went into shock, he started measuring blood pressure, not noticing that the others were waiting for instructions from him. When we focus on practical action, we lose some of our *leadership*, don't we?" The second part of the paraphrase confirms the discovery made by the group (debriefer and learners) and achieves a reinforcing effect. In fact, it is the debriefer who summarizes, acknowledges, and reinforces the individual's discovery that now becomes collective, bringing home an educational result: the learners are understanding that the *leader* should not do, but direct. The same experience is seen from another perspective: "The real voyage of discovery is not to see new worlds, but to change eyes" (Proust).

Saying "correct me if I'm wrong" makes the participants feel that they are the ones leading the process of the discovery dialogue. This restitution by the debriefer of the learners' discoveries in the form of a paraphrase serves to consolidate them, highlighting how they came about from below and not imposed a priori by the debriefer, who in turn reaffirms in this way his role as "facilitator" and not as "managing teacher."

Paraphrasing creates a climate of collaborative relationship between debriefer and learner, who feels accepted and becomes the author of the discovery made about the problem presented and its resolution. In addition, it helps consolidate in the learner the conviction that even if mistakes have been made, the most important thing is what one does with those mistakes because, as Huxley says, "reality is not what happens to us, but what we do with what happens to us."

After the first set of questions, we begin to delve, "funnel," into each topic and each participant, in a circular fashion. As an example, Speech Box 5.5 shows a series of funnel questions on the topic of *leadership*.

Speech Box 5.5 Examples of Sequential Questions to Explore the Leadership Domain

"

Sequential Questions

1. Was there a leader? Who? Why? If not: Can a leaderless team endanger the patient?

2. What did the leader think was happening and what did he/she communicate?

3. Was the team's goal clear to everyone? Was it clearly stated by the leader?

4. Did the leader organize the team? Yes/No, Why? How?

5. Did the leader make decisions alone or were there suggestions? from whom? Why? How did the leader use the suggestions? Why?

6. What requests were made but not heard and/or executed? Why?

7. Was/does the team/staff feel over-or under-utilized? Why?

8. Did the leader regularly re-evaluate the situation? Did he/she do his/her re-evaluation alone or together with his/her team?

9. Did the leader check that his delegations, commands, and instructions were carried out correctly?

10. Was there a change in leadership within the scenario? Why, with whom?

11. Was there conflict between the leaders?

"

Sometimes, to reinforce the discovery result of the individual or group of learners, the debriefer can associate the restructuring paraphrase with an evocative sentence. The technique always consists of using the learner's own words to reformulate the definition of the problem, but this time, rhetorical figures are used that fit the subject and the learner's feelings, to facilitate change, because "before convincing the intellect, it is necessary to touch and prepare the heart" (Pascal).

In the above example, the paraphrase could be completed as follows: "If I understand correctly, correct me if I'm wrong, the *leader* distributed the workloads fairly and managed to converse with his team effectively, but when the patient suddenly went into shock, he started measuring his blood pressure not noticing that the others were waiting for instructions from him. When we focus on a practical thing, we lose some *leadership*, don't we? However, thanks to the nurse reporting the monitor parameters in a timely manner, there were no problems. Every member of the team is the eye and ear of the *leader*."

The feeling you want to evoke is that the team is not composed of simply passive executors, but of effectively vigilant professionals (eyes and ears), who can represent a barrier to any errors or oversights of the *leader*.

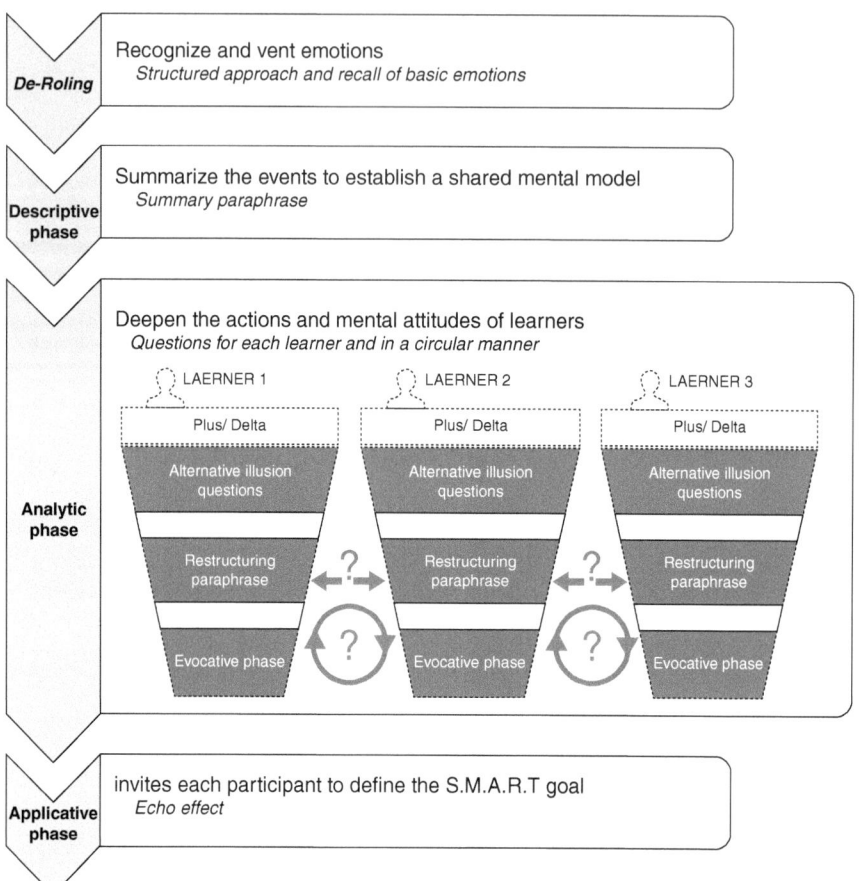

Fig. 5.3 "Funnel" diagram of strategic debriefing

Evocative language can use all rhetorical figures and poetic forms: aphorisms, metaphors, anecdotes, concrete examples, narratives, or counternarratives. This technique is used to create aversion toward attitudes or behaviors that need to be interrupted or changed and attraction toward those reactions that need to be encouraged or increased.

In the analytical phase, the debriefer will be responsible for talking, in turn, with each of the participants while involving the whole team, in a circular way, so that the discovery of one is shared and approved by all (consolidation effect) as illustrated in Fig. 5.3.

Even if a strategic approach is adopted, when the debriefer feels that each of the participants has obtained a result, i.e., has constructively reflected on even one behavior to be improved, he can close the analytical phase and move on to the next one (application phase).

Table 5.2 summarizes, with brief examples, the different styles that can be used in the analytical phase of the debriefing.

Table 5.2   The different styles used in the analytical phase

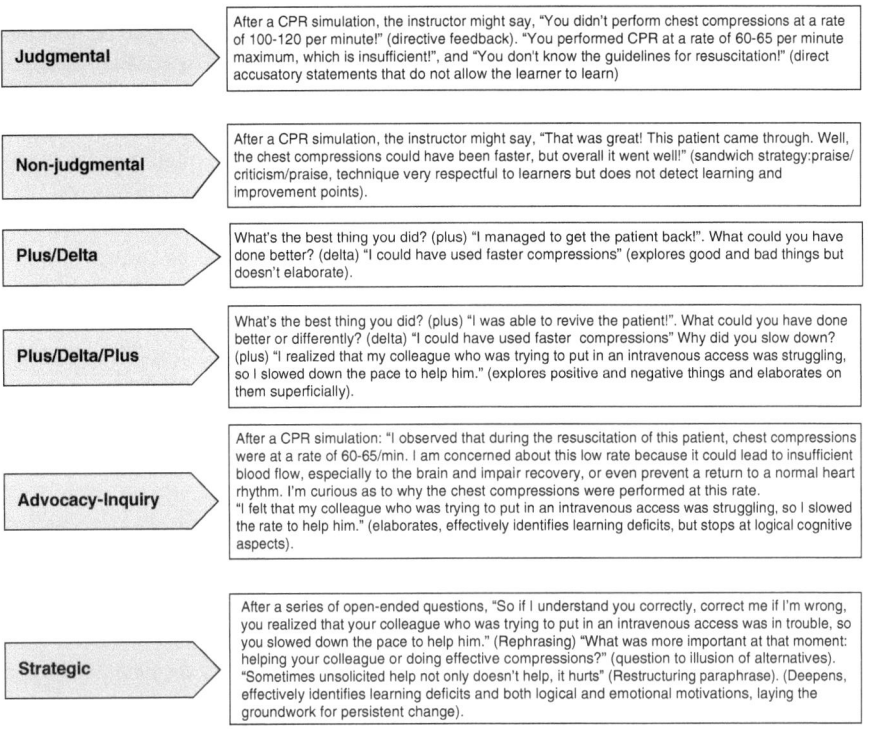

Judgmental	After a CPR simulation, the instructor might say, "You didn't perform chest compressions at a rate of 100-120 per minute!" (directive feedback). "You performed CPR at a rate of 60-65 per minute maximum, which is insufficient!", and "You don't know the guidelines for resuscitation!" (direct accusatory statements that do not allow the learner to learn)
Non-judgmental	After a CPR simulation, the instructor might say, "That was great! This patient came through. Well, the chest compressions could have been faster, but overall it went well!" (sandwich strategy:praise/criticism/praise, technique very respectful to learners but does not detect learning and improvement points).
Plus/Delta	What's the best thing you did? (plus) "I managed to get the patient back!". What could you have done better? (delta) "I could have used faster compressions" (explores good and bad things but doesn't elaborate).
Plus/Delta/Plus	What's the best thing you did? (plus) "I was able to revive the patient!". What could you have done better or differently? (delta) "I could have used faster compressions" Why did you slow down? (plus) "I realized that my colleague who was trying to put in an intravenous access was struggling, so I slowed down the pace to help him." (explores positive and negative things and elaborates on them superficially).
Advocacy-Inquiry	After a CPR simulation: "I observed that during the resuscitation of this patient, chest compressions were at a rate of 60-65/min. I am concerned about this low rate because it could lead to insufficient blood flow, especially to the brain and impair recovery, or even prevent a return to a normal heart rhythm. I'm curious as to why the chest compressions were performed at this rate. "I felt that my colleague who was trying to put in an intravenous access was struggling, so I slowed the rate to help him." (elaborates, effectively identifies learning deficits, but stops at logical cognitive aspects).
Strategic	After a series of open-ended questions, "So if I understand you correctly, correct me if I'm wrong, you realized that your colleague who was trying to put in an intravenous access was in trouble, so you slowed down the pace to help him." (Rephrasing) "What was more important at that moment: helping your colleague or doing effective compressions?" (question to illusion of alternatives). "Sometimes unsolicited help not only doesn't help, it hurts" (Restructuring paraphrase). (Deepens, effectively identifies learning deficits and both logical and emotional motivations, laying the groundwork for persistent change).

5.7   The Application Phase

The concluding or application phase can very briefly summarize the topics covered and lessons learnt, emphasizing their importance in relation to the workplace. It is good to anticipate that the debriefing session is ending, for example, by saying "it's time to end the debriefing session," reminding participants that they are entering the application phase, that is, the phase in which each participant shares what they have learned from the simulation.

5.7.1   In Basic Debriefing

Typically, the debriefer asks each of the participants to say, in turn, the most important thing they learned from the scenario and debriefing and how this will affect their future clinical practice. It is not possible to comment on each other's conclusions at this stage as this very personal process of sharing deserves the utmost respect and listening from everyone.

The typical questions are, "What did you learn? What are you taking home with you? What will you take away from today's scenario for your daily practice? How will you do it?" At the end of the round, the debriefer will also share what he or she learned, to testify, in a meta-communicative way, that from the simulation, everyone learns from each other.

If you have debriefed students or learners who are not experts in the subject matter, it is not uncommon at this point for students to ask for instructional references to study from. Others may express the need to practice a specific procedure several times on a *task trainer*. For this reason, it is advisable for the debriefer to prepare handouts or technical and bibliographical hints in advance explaining the recommendations on the topic of the simulation session and to offer participants who wish to do so the opportunity to study procedures that are not yet well established in more detail in another session. In such cases, the debriefer should also ask himself whether the request for additional teaching tools does not conceal an organizational shortcoming in the students' preliminary preparation for the scenario.

The application phase always ends with the debriefer thanking all learners for their active participation and their efforts to improve their performance.

5.7.2 In Strategic Debriefing

In the application phase, each participant, including the debriefer, any actors, or technicians who attended the session, is asked to share what they have learned, and the typical question in this phase is, "What are you taking home with you?" The answer might be, "I learned that it is important to communicate."

Although at a preliminary observation this could be a good result, in reality, its generic expression hides a shallow and unconvincing approach. In fact, it is comparable to an invitation of the type "So, see you soon?" which usually results in not seeing each other, despite the best intentions. A different kind of invitation would be: "So, see you next Tuesday at 6 o'clock, in Piazza Rossi, for a cup of coffee?" In this second case, the question expresses the concrete and effective intention of the request, which obliges the interlocutor to take an operative decision anyway. In the same way, the debriefer, in order for the application phase to be effective, must ask each of the participants exactly what they are taking home and how this can become a small, but sure, agent of change, necessary so that what was learned in the debriefing is really put into practice. In essence, the learner is asked not only to share what he or she has learned but is prompted to reflect on how the debriefing experience may represent his or her first step toward personal change that may, in turn, result in positive change in his or her clinical work in the hospital. To do this, the debriefer introduces the learners to the technique of SMART goal setting [9]. The goal must be specific (concrete and clear), measurable (defined in terms of observable results), actionable (actually feasible), achievable (based on constraints and resources), and timed (achievable in a given period of time). The debriefer will then ask the question in such a way that the "I'm taking home/I'm personally taking home" responds to the realization of a goal that is SMART, and, in particular, is the smallest step to a truly actionable change that depends solely on the learner (you can't change things that don't depend on us).

If the learner in the application phase is able to define a SMART goal related to what he/she has learned in the scenario, it means that a good strategic debriefing has previously taken place.

For example, usually after a traditional debriefing to the questions "What did you learn? What are you taking home with you?", the learner might answer, "I learned that it is important to communicate using the closed loop method." The strategic debriefer is not satisfied with this answer but invites the learner to delve deeper into their goal and assess whether it is a real (i.e., SMART) goal or a generic assertion.

After a good strategic debriefing, the SMART response might be, "Tomorrow, at the first emergency that happens to me, I will make my request to the nurse by calling him by name, looking him in the eye, and asking for feedback on the action taken." There is no doubt that this definition will more likely lead the learner to effective change because it is based on a stated goal that is dependent on him/her, feasible, measurable, timed, and emotionally internalized, due to the strategic dialogue used during the previous analysis phase.

After all session participants ("teachers" and learners) have participated in the application phase and stated what they have learnt and the resulting SMART personal goals, the debriefer may close the session by thanking everyone and, using evocative language, leave everyone with a suggestion, using a short sentence (aphorism, story, anecdote, quotation) that functions as an anchor and emotional stabilization of the discovery made by the participants (echo effect). For example, if the participants of the session have discovered the value of simulation in their clinical practice, the debriefer could launch an "echo effect" as follows: "There are professionals, the component masters of an orchestra, who spend their professional lives rehearsing and rehearsing several times, only to be able to perform the performance (the concert) once, perfectly and without errors. Other professionals, doctors, claim to perform their single performance perfectly and without error without ever having rehearsed it once before."

Table 5.3 summarizes the basic and advanced strategic debriefing phases.

Table 5.3 Phases in basic and strategic debriefing

	Standard Debriefing	Strategic Debriefing
De-roleing		Analysis of felt emotions
Introduction		
Descriptive phase	Scenario Reconstruction	Scenario Reconstruction Debriefer's summary: experienced and perceived
Analytical phase	Open questions Who, What, When, How Plus/Delta Deepening: Why	Open questions Closed questions to illusion of answer Reformulation - Restructuring Image Agreement with the group Individual and group restructuring
Application phase	From scenario to real life What I have learned What I can do in practice	From scenario to real life What I have learned Objective (SMART) to be pursued Debriefer echo effect

5.8   The Difficult Debriefing

The first prevention of a difficult debriefing is the correct scenario setup. The debriefer must always ensure that the learners are familiar with the simulator and the simulation environment before the scenario begins. For example, a learner who did not understand or was not correctly informed that the respiratory murmur of the manikin may change in accordance with the pathology could create problems within the scenario due to this incompetence, dragging the team off track. Fortunately, in this case, a "last minute" corrective is possible represented by the voice of the manikin itself, guided by the control room, declaring to be asthmatic or, if present, by the action of an actor playing the role of the nurse, who can suggest the maneuver or do it himself. But we don't always have correctives available within the scenario, and so it must be remembered that misunderstandings about the use of the simulator can seriously undermine the debriefing and should therefore be carefully prevented by a good briefing before the scenario.

The explanation of the scenario may, mistakenly, also be oversimplified, as in the case of participants whom the debriefer believes do not need too much explanation because they have had previous simulation experience.

There are also some difficulties that do not depend on the preparation of the scenario and that the debriefer has to deal with. If the debriefer is a beginner, it is very useful to take notes during the scenario and to use cognitive aids, e.g., a checklist, a list of typical questions to ask the participants, or an outline of the debriefing steps and how to proceed.

Among the difficulties of those starting out is how to stay on schedule, and this can be overcome by keeping a clock close by and training yourself to manage the passage of time.

For those starting out in facilitation, it is therefore essential to record and review their sessions together with experienced colleagues who can in turn give feedback or, better still, when and if possible, face a "debriefing of the debriefing" by a very experienced colleague immediately after, or very soon after, the debriefing they have just facilitated.

Particularly difficult, especially for novice or very young debriefers, is the facilitation of older and very experienced participants, or those who hold management positions or who may be their direct superiors in the hospital. Experts are usually reluctant to share their experiences and question them, take it for granted that their practice is the right one, and sometimes even try to take control of the debriefing itself.

It would be desirable if, during a simulation course, the director took care not to expose his younger or inexperienced facilitators to situations such as the one described above.

But the most stressful situation for a non-specifically trained debriefer is when dealing with "difficult learners," such as those who think the simulation is all a game, the overly critical of themselves, the aggressive who heavily criticize others, the "know-it-all," the quiet introverts, etc.

Below are some basic suggestions for getting started with a debriefing where one or more types of difficult participants are present, referring to specialized texts and completion of advanced training courses specific to the topic.

In the vast majority of cases, these are resistant learners, i.e., those who in one way or another resist change induced by simulation.

The brief strategic approach teaches that there are four different types of resistance to change: resistance of the "oppositional" type, the "collaborative" type, the "I want to but I can't" type, and the "I can't collaborate or oppose" type.

It must be remembered that resistances always refer to the behavior and not to the character of the person and that the approach of the strategic debriefer is not to challenge or oppose them, but to use ad hoc created stratagems to exploit them and redirect them to promote change. Any resistance to change is not a characteristic of the individual person but of his or her interaction with the type of change being requested, who is requesting it, and the context and time in which it is being requested.

Oppositional learners are not uncommon, especially among those participants who have been in some way forced to participate in a simulation course, for example, in the case of company courses, or if the participants are colleagues who have previously unresolved conflicts between themselves. This learner tends to disqualify our proposals, pointing out areas of ineffectiveness or inappropriateness, challenges the realism of the scenario, and opposes technical and behavioral suggestions. He often refuses to engage because "it's all a game anyway."

To this category belong also the critics at all costs, the "mister know-it-all" and those who, possessing a rigid personality, have not been able to enter the spirit of the simulation. Oppositional behavior may also be due to fear of being judged and exposing oneself to criticism, especially when dealing with experienced or elderly clinicians. Oppositional behavior may also be due to the debriefer's failure to explain the differences between clinical reality and the realism of the scenario and to persuade participants to behave during the scenario as they would in the real world. In all these cases, the debriefer may experience frustration and annoyance and risk taking it personally, seriously compromising the progress of the debriefing.

The intervention consists in transforming resistance into fulfilment instead of opposition. In this way, the main function of the resistance is cancelled, and it becomes the main engine of change (the technique of "killing the snake with its own venom"). For example, one could thank the oppositional person, telling him or her that "What you see, no one else sees, so I ask you to help me identify the deficiencies that have occurred" and giving him or her a constructive task without entering into the content of the discussion (establishment of a paradoxical double bond). The debriefer in these cases should know how to interrupt and at the same time know how to listen to his oppositional learner with polite firmness.

At the opposite end of the spectrum is the collaborative learner, who enthusiastically welcomes the novelty of the simulation method and always agrees to implement it. The debriefer's first impression is that they are satisfied to have an enthusiastic learner, and this leads to an underestimation of this type of behavior.

In fact, the collaborative participant may take over and influence the course of the discussion. The collaborative participant may tend to overdo it and going further may not go in the desired direction. He or she is a person who creates disorder rather than resistance, and this may interfere with desired personal and group change.

To this category also belongs the histrionic, who, despite not having particular skills, tends to be present at any cost. The strategic debriefer can deal with this type of learner by accepting their collaboration, but at the same time containing it, transforming an oppositional symmetry into a complementary collaborative position. For example, one might say, "Thank you for your valuable contribution, but allow me to go step by step to make sure everyone can keep up...."

The "I would like to but I can't" learner realizes that he/she should change and modify his/her attitude but is unable to do so because he/she does not have the emotional or behavioral resources necessary to implement the change. This may be the case of learners who, at the end of the debriefing, in the application phase, are unable to take home a change project, not because they have not discovered or learned anything but because they have an emotional block or because a change in clinical and behavioral attitudes seems impossible for them to achieve once back in their hospital. In this case, the debriefer will be able to quantify the commitment, helping the learner to offer to take the smallest step compatible with what they feel like doing. Even a single different attitude can be the small snowflake that will generate the avalanche of change in his working environment. If the resistance is mainly due to an emotional block, you will have to work with an emotional language of images rather than a rational logical language.

Finally, the participant can offer resistance such as "I can neither cooperate nor oppose."

The person implementing this type of resistance is usually a rigid person, who appeals to his values and beliefs that he considers incompatible with the change proposed by the simulation scenario.

The debriefer may experience a risky feeling of discouragement in this case and doubt that the learner is "in it or out of it?" or is "unintelligent" and is likely to feel that their learner is "a lost cause," or to think that they are doing it on purpose.

We are dealing with a person with such a strong mental rigidity that it prevents him from coming out of his own vision of reality and to put himself at risk. The technique to use is that of putting oneself in her shoes, entering into her logic, assuming her linguistic codes, and introducing elements into her dysfunctional logical reasoning that do not contradict or disqualify her, but that reorient her toward new directions until she is completely restructured. Open-ended questions and assertions that do not challenge her point of view are essential, so you must first agree and confirm her positions and then add an additional element, such as "If I understand correctly, correct me if I am wrong, your thinking on this subject is this... so you will certainly agree that we could also add...." It's like moving politely and cautiously into some stranger's home. The debriefer should also always keep in mind that the more rigid a person is, the more fragile they are.

5.9   How to Evaluate the Debriefing

Like all activities, debriefing should be done regularly and, at first, under supervision. In principle, good debriefing can already be easily recognized if:

- There is respectful discussion in the group
- The debriefer doesn't talk too much and facilitates discussion rather than lecturing
- Everyone in the group is involved
- Everyone, even the shy, contributes and doesn't feel judged
- "Boisterous" participants are "contained" with respect
- The discussion is more about what the participants are interested in than what the debriefer set out to discuss
- The participants learn from each other
- Videos are introduced and used appropriately
- Appropriate and inappropriate technical skills and strategies for improvement were discussed
- Aspects of communication and strategies for improvement were discussed
- In the end, no one felt disappointed in themselves
- All participants learned at least one thing about themselves and left the session vowing to reflect on what had learned again by incorporating it into their future clinical practice

However, for more precise assessment and to help the debriefer to receive adequate feedback on their progress, a number of assessment methodologies have been described [10–12], but the best known and most widely used methods to facilitate debriefing assessment are the *Objective Structured Assessment of Debriefing* (OSAD) [13] and the *Debriefing Assessment for Simulation in Healthcare* (DASH) [14].

The OSAD (Table 5.4) evaluates the performance of the facilitator in a fairly detailed way and can be used not only as an absolute score, but, in our opinion, also in a more dynamic way, to check the learning path and the acquisition of the various skills of the learner-debriefer. The OSAD assigns a score from 1 (poor performance) to 5 (very good performance) for each of the debriefer's basic activities:

1. Approach: evaluates the way in which the facilitator leads the debriefing session, his/her level of enthusiasm and positivity, his/her interest in establishing and maintaining a rapport with the participants, and his/her ability to end the session on a positive note

Table 5.4 OSAD score

	1	2	3	4	5
Approach	Judgmental comparison		Tries to establish rapport with participants but is either too critical or too informal		Establishes and maintains rapport throughout the session. Uses a non-judgmental but honest approach, creating a psychologically safe environment
Establish a suitable learning environment	Participant expectations are not clear or clarified, there are no rules for how to participate		Explains the purpose of the debriefing but does not clarify participants' expectations		Explains the purpose of the debriefing and clarifies participants' expectations and goals at the beginning of the debriefing
Commitment to participants	Purely didactic, it is aimed primarily at those who intervene in the discussion, not involving those who remain passive		Participants are involved in the discussion, but mainly through closed questions, those who remain more passive are not involved.		Encourage participation with open-ended questions. Invite everyone to participate in the discussion
Reflection	No recognition of participants' reactions or the emotional impact of the experience		Asks participants how they feel, but does not fully explore their reaction to the event		Fully explores participants' reactions, and appropriately confronts those who are dissatisfied
Reaction	No possibility of self-analysis, participants are not asked what really happened during the scenario		The debriefer mentions some description of the events but with little self-reflection by the participants.		Encourage participants to do some self-reflection on the incident using a step-by-step approach.
Analysis	The reasons for and consequences of actions are not examined.		The facilitator (not the participants) explores the reasons and consequences of actions but doesn't offer the opportunity to relate them to previous experiences.		Help participants explore their actions and the consequences of their actions by identifying specific examples and relating them to previous experiences.
Diagnosis	No feedback on team skills, does not identify performance deficiencies or provide positive reinforcement		Feedback is provided only on technical skills, it focuses only on mistakes and not on the behavior that caused them.		Provides objective feedback on both technical and team skills, identifies positive behaviors as well as performance shortcomings, highlighting in particular behaviors that can be changed
Application	Offers no opportunity for participants to identify strategies for future improvement or to consolidate learning points		Discussion of learning points and strategies for improvement, but lacks application to future practice		Reinforces key points identified by participants and highlights how strategies for improvement can be applied in future clinical practice

2. Creating the enabling environment for learning: assesses the ability to introduce the session by explaining to the learners what is expected of them during the debriefing, emphasizing the basic rules of confidentiality and respect for others and encouraging participants to identify their own learning objectives
3. Participant engagement: assesses the ability to actively engage all participants during the discussion, asking open-ended questions to explore their thoughts, and using silence to encourage their contribution without intervening most of the time to ensure deep rather than superficial learning
4. Reflection: ability to induce self-reflection on the events that occurred during the scenario step by step in a factual manner, clarifying each technical-clinical topic from the beginning, to allow (the) reflection of all participants toward the analysis and application phase, linking them to previous experiences
5. Reaction: assesses the ability to determine how much the simulation experience had an emotional impact on participants
6. Analysis: assesses the ability to stimulate the cognitive processes that drove participants' actions, using specific examples of observable behaviors to allow the participant to make sense of the simulation session
7. Diagnosis: evaluates the ability to enable the participant to identify performance deficits and strategies for improvement, highlighting only those behaviors that can be improved or changed and then giving a structured feedback and objective of the simulation session
8. Application: assesses the ability to summarize the learning points and strategies for improvement that were identified by participants during the debriefing and how these can be applied to change their future clinical practice

The DASH is a self-assessment questionnaire which the debriefer can fill in to assess himself, but there is also a version in which the trainees assess their debriefer. Of both questionnaires, there is an extended form (23 items) and a short form (6 items) which require different filling in times and can therefore be used in different situations. Table 5.5 shows the questionnaire of the debriefer's self-assessment.

Table 5.5 DASH rating scale [5]

SCORE / DESCRIPTOR	1 Definitely ineffective/harmful	2 Constantly ineffective/poor	3 Mostly ineffective/poor	4 Fairly effective/ medium	5 Mostly effective/good	6 Mostly effective/ very good	7 Extremely effective/ very good	SCORE
1. Creating an engaging learning environment								
A. The debriefer introduced himself, described the simulation environment, what would be expected during the activity, introduced the learning objectives, and discussed confidentiality and roles.								
B. The debriefer explained the strengths and weaknesses of the simulation and what participants could do to get the most out of the simulation experience.								
C. The debriefer took care of the necessary logistical details, such as the location of restrooms, food availability, and schedules.								
D. The debriefer expressed a commitment to respect the participants by welcoming them to share their thoughts and questions about the upcoming simulation and debriefing and reassured them that they would not be judged.								
2. Maintaining an engaging learning environment								
A. The debriefer clarified the purpose of the debriefing, what was expected of the participants, and his role in the debriefing								
B. The debriefer acknowledged learners' concerns about realism and helped them to overcome them								
C. The debriefer expressed respect for the participants.								
D. The focus was on learning and not on embarrassing people who make mistakes.								
E. Participants were able to share thoughts and emotions without fear of being judged.								
3. Organized debriefing								
A. The conversation progressed logically, rather than jumping from one point to another.								
B. Towards the beginning of the debriefing, participants were encouraged to share their genuine reactions to the case(s) and the debriefer seemed to take their observations seriously								
C. During the analytic phase, the debriefer helped participants analyze their actions and thought processes as they reviewed the case(s).								
D. At the end of the debriefing, there was a synthesis phase in which the debriefer helped connect observations and relate the case(s) to ways in which participants could improve their future clinical practice.								
4. Ability to engage in discussion								
A. The debriefer used concrete examples - not just abstract or generalized comments - to get participants to reflect on their performance.								
B. The debriefer's point of view was clear; participants did not have to guess what the debriefer was thinking.								
C. The debriefer listened and made people feel heard by trying to include everyone, paraphrasing, and using nonverbal actions such as eye contact and nodding, etc.								
D. Debriefer used video or recorded data to support analysis and learning								
E. If someone became upset during the debriefing, the debriefer was respectful and constructive in trying to help and address it.								
5. Ability to identify and explore deficits in learner performance								
A. Participants received concrete feedback on their individual performance or that of their team based on the debriefer's honest and accurate point of view								
B. The debriefer helped to explore what participants were thinking or trying to achieve at key moments.								
6. Aid to doctors in training								
A. Debriefer helped participants learn how to improve weak areas or how to repeat a good performance								
B. The debriefer was knowledgeable and used this knowledge to help the participants see how to get good results in the future.								
C. The debriefer made sure the discussion covered important topics.								

References

1. Kim, J., Neilipovitz, D., Cardinal, P., & Chiu, M. (2009). A comparison of global rating scale and checklist scores in the validation of an evaluation tool to assess performance in the resuscitation of critically ill patients during simulated emergencies (abbreviated as "CRM simulator study IB"). *Simulation in Healthcare, 4*(1), 6–16.
2. Franc, J. M., Verde, M., Gallardo, A. R., Carenzo, L., & Ingrassia, P. L. (2017). An Italian version of the Ottawa Crisis Resource Management Global Rating Scale: A reliable and valid tool for assessment of simulation performance. *Internal and Emergency Medicine, 12*(5), 651–656.
3. van de Hart, O. (1983). *Rituals in psychotherapy: Transition and continuity.* Irvington.
4. Fanning, R. M., & Gaba, D. M. (2007). The role of debriefing in simulation-based learning. *Simulation in Healthcare, 2*(2), 115–125.
5. Center for Medical Simulation. (2018). Retrieved from https://harvardmedsim.org/
6. Rudolph, J. W., Simon, R., Dufresne, R. L., & Raemer, D. B. (2006). There's no such thing as "nonjudgmental" debriefing: A theory and method for debriefing with good judgment. *Simulation in Healthcare, 1*(1), 49–55.
7. Eppich, W., & Cheng, A. (2015). Promoting Excellence and Reflective Learning in Simulation (PEARLS): Development and rationale for a blended approach to health care simulation debriefing. *Simulation in Healthcare, 10*(2), 106–115.
8. Nardone, G., & Salvini, A. (2004). *The strategic dialogue.* Ponte alle Grazie.
9. Doran, G. T. (1981). There's a S.M.A.R.T. way to write management's goals and objectives. *Management Review, 70*(11), 35–36.
10. Bradley, C. S., & Dreifuerst, K. T. (2016). Pilot testing the debriefing for meaningful learning evaluation scale. *Clinical Simulation in Nursing, 12*(7), 277–280.
11. Reed, S. J. (2012). Debriefing experience scale: Development of a tool to evaluate the student learning experience in debriefing. *Clinical Simulation in Nursing, 8*(6), e211–e217.
12. Tosterud, R., Petzäll, K., Wangensteen, S., & Hall-Lord, M. L. (2015). Cross-cultural validation and psychometric testing of the questionnaire: Debriefing experience scale. *Clinical Simulation in Nursing, 11*(1), 27–34.
13. Arora, S., Ahmed, M., Paige, J., Nestel, D., Runnacles, J., Hull, L., Darzi, A., & Sevdalis, N. (2012). Objective structured assessment of debriefing: Bringing science to the art of debriefing in surgery. *Annals of Surgery, 256*(6), 982–988.
14. Brett-Fleegler, M., Rudolph, J., Eppich, W., Monuteaux, M., Fleegler, E., Cheng, A., & Simon, R. (2012). Debriefing assessment for simulation in healthcare: Development and psychometric properties. *Simulation in Healthcare, 7*(5), 288–294.

Appendixes

Appendix A: Debriefing with Regular Staff

Scenario Title
A busy night
   Neonatal resuscitation in the delivery room

Participants and Roles
MICHELA: debriefer
GIULIA: neonatologist
ALICE: nursery physician
SABRINA: midwife
DANIELA: Neonatal Intensive Care Unit (NICU) nurse

Simulation Site
In the simulation center

Scenario Description
The scenario took place in the delivery room where *Alice*, a nursery physician, and *Sabrina*, a midwife, were involved in resuscitating a pale and atonic baby just extracted from an urgent caesarean section for placental abruption. In the course of the scenario, *Giulia*, neonatologist, was called to their aid, arriving accompanied by *Daniela*, neonatal intensive care nurse.

The participants are healthcare professionals, all from the same hospital, and play the same professional role in the scenario as they do in life.

Debriefing

De-roling
Immediately after finishing the scenario, as they leave the simulation room, the debriefer facilitates de-roling, trying to get the scenario participants to express their emotions.

Speaker	Dialogue		Comments
MICHELA *Debriefer*	*How are you feeling?*	●—→	The first crucial moment in which the debriefer deals with the emotions of the scenario participants is the reaction phase. This phase, in addition to serving the learners to decompress and step out of the role they played during the scenario, is very useful for the debriefer to understand the emotional state of each of the learners, which will inevitably, if not handled appropriately, reflect negatively in turn on the debriefing discussion and the learning itself. The strategic model considers this phase a real first phase of emotional deepening, preliminary to the debriefing itself The typical question in this phase is "How do you feel?" or "How did you feel during the scenario?" In this case, the debriefer asked an open-ended question to all participants, without specifying anyone in particular. It would have been better to address the question to each of the participants, starting with the one who entered first, or the most inexperienced, or the shyest, if you want to avoid that the most charismatic could influence the other shy ones with his answer. Notice how having addressed his question in a generic way without directing it to anyone in particular, the answers were evasive, not pertinent to the question, and how, above all, not all the participants answered, but only some of them
GIULIA *Neonatologist*	*I feel a widespread feeling of anxiety, but I felt completely immersed in the simulation, and actually it seemed to me to be there around the neonatal resuscitation bed, just as if it was real.*		
SABRINA *Midwife*	*We experienced a scene similar to the one we experience every day in our clinical practice*		
ALICE *Nursery physician*	*It was realistic.*		

Speaker	Dialogue		Comments
MICHELA *Debriefer*	*Sabrina, what was the first emotion you felt, in a word?*	●—►	From here on, the debriefer addresses each of the participants, and as can be seen, the dialogue is much more orderly and the responses more to the point. The debriefer goes in search of each participant's emotion. If the answer is evasive, it is necessary to insist, repeating the question and trying to get a description of an emotion
SABRINA *Midwife*	*(agitation)* *How about you, Daniela?*		
DANIELA *NICU Nurse*	*Eh yes, the same thing for me too: anxiety, because when the call of the delivery team arrives, you feel the same feeling. There is a baby who is sick, and you have to intervene; you have to do many things well all together. In this simulation, I was careful with just the right amount of anxiety.*		
MICHELA *Debriefer*	*"Right" anxiety, good, thank you. And you, ALICE, what feelings did you have?*		
ALICE *Nursery physician*	*The scenario was very realistic and however experiencing it maybe repeatedly helps you better manage the anxiety that can happen to you in reality.*		
MICHELA *Debriefer*	*Yes Alice, but I asked you to express your feeling. What emotion did you feel?*	●—►	This is the correct way to invite the participant to answer the question posed without rambling. It is important at this stage that everyone expresses their emotions and reserves the right to speak and comment on the scenario only later, in the analytical phase
ALICE *Nursery physician*	*I had some anxiety too.*		

Speaker	Dialogue		Comments
MICHELA *Debriefer*	*So, if I understand you correctly, correct me if I'm wrong, it seems to me that anxiety was the emotion that prevailed for all the team members. Shall we try to quickly understand why? Let's start with Giulia. What do you think generated your anxiety: the fear of not being sufficiently prepared to handle the situation or that the worst could happen?*	●—▶	Through the debriefer's illusion of alternative questions, the participant discovers that her "anxiety" was actually "fear." The participant's discovery is then reframed (restructured) by the debriefer to consolidate the discovery Restructuring is a technique of strategic dialogue. Restructuring means recoding a person's perception of reality without changing the meaning of things but changing their structure. In practice, you change the frame, but by changing the frame, the point of view, and therefore the perception, the meaning itself will change. This is because an event, looked at within different contexts and from different perspectives, itself changes its value
GIULIA Neonatologist	*I'm afraid of not being prepared enough!*		
MICHELA *Debriefer*	*Thanks Giulia! We'll see why you felt this sensation in the analytical phase.*		
GIULIA Neonatologist	*Yes, great!*		
MICHELA *Debriefer*	*Thanks Giulia!* *You, Sabrina, mentioned before your agitation: can you better define this feeling?*		
SABRINA *Midwife*	*In fact, if I think about it I was worried because I was afraid of not being able to do it.*		
MICHELA *Debriefer*	*Were you afraid you weren't up to the task, didn't feel prepared enough, or were you afraid of being judged in this scenario?*	●—▶	With this illusion of alternative question, the debriefer tries to investigate the roots of the participant's fear, who is finally able to express the true emotion he had inside. This will serve the participant himself to decompress and the debriefer to understand the participant's state of mind, and this can be very useful during the analytical phase of debriefing

Speaker	Dialogue		Comments
SABRINA *Midwife*	*No, being a midwife and having to deal with two neonatologists and a nurse specialized in neonatology, I felt little able to help. There, it was fear of not being adequate!*		
MICHELA *Debriefer*	*Well Sabrina, we'll go into this in more detail in the debriefing, for now thank you!*		
	Alice, you also talked about "a bit of anxiety": could you better define this feeling?	●→	The same in-depth methodology is addressed to each of the participants
ALICE *Nursery physician*	*The scenario was very realistic, and maybe that's why I was afraid of being judged by those who were watching us in the control room. Maybe it happened only at the beginning, then I immersed myself in the clinical case, and I forgot to be in a simulation.*	●→	The reference to the fear of being judged by the instructors in the initial phase of the scenario may suggest some problem with the realism of the scenario or the way it is presented during the briefing. Without going into it, the debriefer will note and memorize this aspect, which may come up during the later analytical phase. The debriefer may also feel that the scenario was not programmed realistically enough in the design phase and will discuss this with the other instructors at the end of the simulation session
MICHELA *Debriefer*	*So, if I have understood well, and correct me if I'm wrong, you were afraid of being judged.*		
ALICE *Nursery physician*	*Yes, correct, at least during the initial phase of the scenario.*		
MICHELA *Debriefer*	*As you said, however, it happened just at the beginning, and thereafter you immersed yourself in the clinical case, forgetting that you were in a simulation. Do you know the ancient Japanese Koan? "The fear of not being good enough is a weapon that allows me to climb one step higher"*		It is quite clear that the initial fear was easily overcome by the participant. The debriefer decided to reframe the participant's feeling by using a catchphrase

Speaker	Dialogue		Comments
MICHELA *Debriefer*	*Thanks Alice! What about you Daniela? Can you tell us why you mentioned anxiety?*		
DANIELA *NICU Nurse*	*I am apprehensive in life and I have an anxious character.*		
MICHELA *Debriefer*	*Yes okay, but could you describe more specifically how you felt during this scenario? Was it a positive, activating anxiety, or was it a negative, "resource blocking" anxiety?*		
DANIELA *NICU Nurse*	*Exactly as in real life, it was a sort of "activating anxiety", with that right amount of adrenaline-fueled anxiety that helps you solve serious cases and act promptly in emergencies!*		
MICHELA *Debriefer*	*Thank you, Daniela! Very good! You are absolutely right, anxiety and fear accompany us in emergencies, and, if they don't overpower us but we know how to manage them, they can be considered a resource and not a limitation.* *We delved into our emotions and found that we all had some fear, albeit of different things. Certainly, during the debriefing, we will have an opportunity, if you will, to find out whether and how much these emotions influenced our clinical behavior or not.* *Thank you, everyone. Now let's head to the briefing room to do our debriefing on the scenario we just experienced.*	●━▶	The de-roling is over. By summarizing everyone's emotions, the debriefer finds consensus among the group and checks if he/she has understood correctly. Awareness of emotions is a cornerstone of change. Becoming aware of the emotional experience and being able to verbalize it provides access to the adaptive information and action tendency of each emotion. Once a person gets in touch with their "feeling," they can more easily connect to their needs (in this case learning needs) and motivate themselves to meet them "There is nothing in the intellect that is not first in the senses" (Thomas Aquinas): a good reaction phase (de-roling) paves the way for a good debriefing!

Introduction

Speaker	Dialogue	Comments
MICHELA *Debriefer*	*Well, now let's start the debriefing. I remind you that there will be no judgments, criticism, or blame, nothing discussed will leave this room; we will try to speak one at a time without overlapping. I will guide you through three different phases: a first phase of description of what happened, in which we will describe what you saw and what happened; the second phase of analysis, in which we will try to understand what happened from different perspectives; and a third phase of synthesis, in which we will discover the application part of this experience, that is, what we learned.*	

Descriptive Phase

Speaker	Dialogue		Comments
MICHELA *Debriefer*	*Let's try to reconstruct what happened. Can you give me a description of the scenario? Sabrina, would you like to start?*	●—→	The debriefer asks Sabrina to make the description of the event for two reasons: first of all, she is the one who entered the scenario first together with Alice and, second, to avoid the "hierarchy" effect, i.e., that the leader, the doctor who entered at the beginning with her, takes the floor and influences the following description
SABRINA *Midwife*	*Alice and I were at the nursery; we received a phone call informing us about the birth of a critical baby; we noticed that the newborn presented pale cyanosis and is bradycardic, and so we called the neonatal intensive care unit (NICU) to look for help, and in fact Giulia, the NICU doctor, arrived at first, and then another call was necessary to activate the specialized nurse.*		
ALICE *Nursery physician*	*I probably made a mistake from the beginning because, since a critical situation was foreseen, we would have done better to call the whole team immediately.*		

Speaker	Dialogue		Comments
MICHELA *Debriefer*	*Thanks Alice, we'll see this better later in the analysis phase [a]. Coming back to the description of what happened, Giulia, when you arrived what did you see? [b]*	●──▶	[a] The debriefer interrupts Alice because she was anticipating a reflection regarding the analytic phase in the descriptive phase. This should be avoided in order not to generate confusion and to accustom participants to an orderly and structured discussion When a participant anticipates a phase, it is important to enhance his intervention and direct it to the right phase so that it can occupy the right space and time for reflection For example, you can say, "this thing you said is too important to deal with now, we'll pick it up later," or "let's finish the description tour and then get back to you." The important thing is that the debriefer doesn't neglect the participant and remembers to engage them in the appropriate phase It is always useful to remember that the order of the debriefing phases is functional to an orderly discussion for maximum profit where the order is given by the debriefer but the content is put by the participants [b] Giulia's opinion is asked because as the leader of the situation, she can give a different reading or add details

Speaker	Dialogue		Comments
GIULIA *Neonatologist*	*When I arrived, there was already a critical situation: Alice was at the head of the newborn baby and was ventilating him, and Sabrina was auscultating him and was helping in the first rescue maneuvers and was positioning the pulse oxymeter. So, I stood at the newborn's head and started to ventilate him; in the meantime, Alice started to listen to his heart rate that was below 100, but also below 60. We continued to ventilate him according to the guidelines and started cardiac massage. Based on the clinical conditions, we then decided to intubate him, and in the meantime, we called the neonatal intensive care unit for help. The nurse immediately came, and with her help, we continued the resuscitation maneuvers.*		
MICHELA *Debriefer*	*Do you agree with the description? Do you want to complete or add something? Daniela, do you have anything to add? You were the last who arrived.*	●→	Before concluding the descriptive phase, the debriefer makes sure that he has heard from everyone; no one should escape, or at least he makes sure that everyone agrees with the description of the event. The debriefer calls Daniela into question because, being the last to enter the scenario, she may have perceived and seen a different picture of the situation from, for example, the participant who entered first. In addition, the last to enter the scenario is usually able to see not only the clinical aspects but also those relating to team behavior (e.g., what the team members were doing when they entered the simulation room), whereas the first to enter, and perhaps alone in the simulation room, will be led to observe only the patient

Speaker	Dialogue		Comments
DANIELA *NICU Nurse*	*When I arrived, there was already a team that was practicing resuscitation, and I had not been told anything. I asked Giulia (neonatologist) what to do, and she gave me precise instructions about the drugs, and I took care of it. At a certain point, on the basis of the parameters Giulia was asking us, we were undecided whether or not to continue resuscitation. Then, Giulia decided to continue, and we went on.* *As Daniela speaks, the other female colleagues nod, confirming the description just given.*		
MICHELA *Debriefer*	*If I have understood correctly, it was an asphyxiated child who was promptly resuscitated, but at some point, you posed the question of whether to continue resuscitation. Have I understood that correctly? Do you agree with that?*	●→	The debriefer summarized the descriptive phase, which serves to make each participant in the scenario understand the experience and the point of view of the others: in this way, the students learn that there is not just one reality, but many realities depending on the points of observation that the various participants have during the scenario Moreover, by using the same language as his pupils, according to the method of strategic dialogue, the debriefer bypasses their possible resistance
ALL	*(Nodding and confirming)*		

Analytic Phase

Speaker	Dialogue		Comments
MICHELA *Debriefer*	*Well, then, we can move on to the analysis phase. Alice, earlier when I interrupted you, you were reflecting on telephone communication, what did you mean by that?*	●→	The debriefer starts the analysis phase from Alice, whom he had previously interrupted during the descriptive phase (see above)

Speaker	Dialogue		Comments
ALICE *Nursery physician*	*Yes, I was thinking that I probably made a mistake because, since a critical situation had been foreseen, I would have been better off immediately alerting the whole neonatal intensive care team, and I could have spent a few more seconds to better explain the criticality of the situation when they arrived.*		
MICHELA *Debriefer*	*Alice is telling us that she could have spent a few more seconds to better explain the criticality of the situation when the NICU team arrived. Daniela, what do you say?*	●→	The debriefer already knew Alice's answer because she had anticipated it earlier, so he repeats it in the same words to evoke the echo effect and asks the others to confirm what Alice experienced
DANIELA *NICU Nurse*	*DANIELA (NURSE): yes, in fact, my initial anxiety was also due to the fact that I didn't know what situation awaited me.*	●→	Return among participants the emotions they themselves reported in de-roling. It is important at this stage of analysis to observe the effect of those emotions on behavior and perceived effectiveness of clinical behaviors The emotional involvement of the participants in the simulation is an indicator of the success of the simulation: we are simulating but the emotions are real
ALICE *Nursery physician*	*In my opinion, at the beginning, we should have immediately pre-alerted the second team; we should have warned them that a "critical" baby was going to be born, and right from the phone call, even if it was brief, we could have told them what it was about; in this way, the neonatal resuscitation team would have already known what was waiting for them, and probably two of them would have arrived right from the first call.*		
MICHELA *Debriefer*	*Do you all agree?*		
ALL	*Yes (Nodding)*		

Speaker	Dialogue		Comments
MICHELA *Debriefer*	*If I understand you correctly, the fact that they went up one at a time was a problem and caused you to lose time, so how could you do it differently next time?*	●—→	Once the critical point has been identified and analyzed, the debriefer asks what concrete action could be taken to improve the situation
ALICE *Nursery physician*	*In fact, every time someone arrives, it is difficult to understand what he/she is talking about as far as it is clear to you; I found myself doing the summary twice: when Giulia arrived then when Daniela came up, probably next time, I will dedicate a few minutes more to the telephone communication, and I will ask my nurse to support me in this.*		
MICHELA *Debriefer*	*I guess to have understood, correct me if I'm wrong, that there was a criticality in communicating the situation: what principle of CRM reminds us what to do in cases like these?*	●—→	The debriefer also introduces a reminder of CRM theory so that it is the participants themselves who identify the CRM principles most suited to the criticality highlighted
DANIELA *NICU Nurse*	*In my opinion "anticipate and plan," with the meaning also of preparing colleagues to what they will face.*		
SABRINA *Midwife*	*It also reminds me of the principle of "asking for help early on."*		
ALICE *Nursery physician*	*Perhaps we were hasty in our call and didn't think it through.*		
MICHELA *Debriefer*	*Then, what would you do differently if you had to redo the scenario?*		
SABRINA *Midwife*	*I would invite Alice to stop for a moment and think about who to call, and once the help has arrived, I would suggest a small briefing before starting.*		
MICHELA *Debriefer*	*Basically, you would try to "spend a little time first, to gain a lot more time later." Napoleon was used to say: "as I am in a hurry, I go very slowly"…*		The debriefer is using an aphorism to better consolidate what the group has discovered and learned

Speaker	Dialogue		Comments
SABRINA *Midwife*	*Yes, certainly.*		
ALL	*(Nodding)*		
MICHELA *Debriefer*	*Let's move on to another point: was there a leader in the situation?*	●—▶	The debriefer, having noticed that all his students have discovered something that they will most likely "take home" in the application phase, decides to close this first trace and move on to analyze another possible criticality
DANIELA *NICU Nurse*	*In my opinion, yes, it was Giulia; I related with her because she is the doctor I usually work with in team in real life, and then when I arrived, I found her at the head of the newborn, and, in my opinion, at the head, there is the leader, and so I related with her immediately, and I asked what I had to do and what had happened.*		
MICHELA *Debriefer*	*Okay, thank you, Daniela. Was it like that for the others? Did you recognize Julia as the leader of the situation because she was at the head of the infant?*	●—▶	The debriefer asks this question in order to make explicit to the group who was the perceived leader and to verify if the impression initially reported by Daniela, who saw Giulia as the leader, is shared by all
SABRINA *Midwife*	*Yes, maybe yes, we have taken for granted that who is in the lead is the leader. In fact, Giulia always gave clear information; she said who had to do what, she made precise requests, she took important decisions like the one to intubate the newborn, and she asked me to give her all the material.*		
ALL	*(Nodding)*		
MICHELA *Debriefer*	*Okay. Giulia, did you feel like you were the leader of the situation?*	●—▶	It is important to check whether the leader recognized by all others felt like "taking on" this role, i.e., whether he managed it consciously and to the best of his potential

Speaker	Dialogue		Comments
GIULIA *Neonatologist*	*Yes, I realized that I assumed the leadership; it comes naturally to me; I worked as I always do in the neonatal intensive care unit. Now, thinking back, all the guidelines of neonatal resuscitation come to my mind, and I think that the distribution of roles was not perfect, that is, when I arrived, I should have exactly said "I am the head and I am the leader of the situation," and so it should have been clear to everybody what I was doing; instead, I took it for granted, and I didn't verbalize it. I could have assigned each team member a role and given them specific tasks, so there would have been a better distribution of roles.*		
MICHELA *Debriefer*	*Do you agree? What do you say? Have you been assigned a role?*	●➤	The debriefer asks the group to confirm what the leader has analyzed as critical. It is essential that the group itself gives feedback, also because in this way, observations and perceptions experienced by all can emerge
ALICE *Nursery physician*	*Giulia was a good leader, at least I felt she was.*		
DANIELA *NICU Nurse*	*In fact, there wasn't an explicit distribution of roles, but considering that we have been working together for years, it was taken for granted.*		
SABRINA *Midwife*	*I think we were caught up in the hurry to assist as soon as possible the critical newborn in front of us.*		
MICHELA *Debriefer*	*So, if I understood correctly, Giulia was the leader because she was at the head of the newborn, she always gave clear information, she distributed the workloads, and she took decisions, but maybe she could have made the roles of the team members more explicit. Giulia do you agree?*	●➤	The debriefer proposes a summary of what has been said so far, using the tool of paraphrasing

Speaker	Dialogue		Comments
GIULIA *Neonatologist*	*Yes, it's just like that. The fact is that we work together in real life, so we played in the scenario the roles we usually play in real life.*		
MICHELA *Debriefer*	*What if you didn't know each other? What could you do to work well together as a really close team?*	●→	The debriefer elaborates, generalizing the specific case
ALICE *Nursery physician*	*First of all, we could have better anticipated the situation by explaining it on the phone, and in any case we could have dedicated some time to the arrival of the second team to think together about what to do.*		
GIULIA *Neonatologist*	*I could have introduced myself at my arrival, before starting the maneuvers on the baby.*		
SABRINA *Midwife*	*We practically already knew who would be the leader, because we know each other, but in case we were a not close team, we should have introduced ourselves.*		
GIULIA *Neonatologist*	*A good method is to call each other by name, reading it on the card, for example, you could say: "Daniela prepare the adrenaline" or "Alice put the COV."*		
MICHELA *Debriefer*	*Calling each other by name sounds like a great idea; is there anything else we could do?* *I don't know…* *What am I doing with you now?* *You're looking at me!*		
	Sure Sabrina, do you think I can get your attention better if I look away while I'm talking, or if I look into your eyes?	●→	The debriefer asks an alternative illusion question, to emphasize the importance of nonverbal communication

Speaker	Dialogue		Comments
SABRINA *Midwife*	*Certainly, when you look into my eyes.*		
MICHELA *Debriefer*	*Do you all agree?*		
ALL	*(Nodding)*		
MICHELA *Debriefer*	*Let's remember the value of nonverbal communication: looking into each other's eyes activates mutual attention and makes communication more effective and efficient. Do you agree?*		
ALL	*(They nod)*	●—→	The debriefer judges that the participants have explored the key issues and, although she knows that there are still other points to be analyzed, is satisfied and stops the analysis phase. It is not always possible, often for reasons of time, to cover every single step of the simulation in an exhaustive way, but it is important to choose carefully which points to cover well. Unless the participants themselves request it, it may often be sufficient to go into detail on only the two or three most significant points. The important thing is that the deepening has met the educational needs of the participants and that they have recognized the points to be improved. In the specific case of this scenario, the topic of "when to discontinue resuscitation" was left unresolved, and the team seemed to lack complete agreement. If the debriefer does not want to miss the opportunity to discuss this important technical topic, he can bring it up again at the end of the debriefing, after the application phase. For example, he could say: "I noticed that some of you expressed some doubts at the beginning of the descriptive phase about the advisability of suspending the resuscitation maneuvers. This seems to me an important topic but one that did not come up from any of you during the analytical phase, but if you would like, now that the debriefing is over, we can take a few more minutes to go over together the guidelines outlining when to discontinue neonatal resuscitation"

Application Phase

Speaker	Dialogue		Comments
MICHELA *Debriefer*	*Now that we have concluded the analysis phase, let's try to draw the lines of what we have been able to learn from this simulation and this debriefing. Let's do it by answering this question: "What do I take home?"*	●—▶	The debriefer begins the synthesis phase, also known as the application phase, in which the concepts treated in the analytical phase are taken up with the intention of transposing them into one's own clinical practice
SABRINA *Midwife*	*I definitely should have worked better on communication, when I asked for the telephone intervention to them, so I definitely need to work more on communication.*		
MICHELA *Debriefer*	*Sabrina, can you tell us the most important thing you learned? And that you're going to put into practice tomorrow when you go back to work? [28]*	●—▶	Sabrina had been generic; the debriefer stimulates her to find a SMART goal to take home that is not generic but can apply concretely to her work context
SABRINA *Midwife*	*If I have a phone call, I will try to specify better what is going on, I will be more careful also in giving some more explanation, and I will also make a more direct request to my colleagues, making explicit that I expect both doctor and nurse to intervene. I will also call my colleagues by name and look them in the eye!*		
MICHELA *Debriefer*	*Well, thank you, Sabrina, it seems to me like a nice commitment, which depends exclusively on you, so I'm sure you'll be able to accomplish it. What are you taking home, Alice?*	●—▶	The debriefer calls each of the participants by name, so as not to exclude anyone and because being called by name activates involvement, including emotional involvement
ALICE *Nursery physician*	*I take home the importance of simulation, in the sense that the situation experienced and tried in simulation will help me face the same situation if it will happen in reality. If I have experienced it, it will be more likely that I will be able to reproduce it!*		

Speaker	Dialogue		Comments
MICHELA *Debriefer*	*So, Alice, if you could describe a SMART goal, i.e., specific, measurable, actionable, achievable, and timed, that you take home … what would it be? Try describing something specific and not general.*	●—▶	The SMART objective means that an objective should be specific (concrete and clear), measurable (defined in terms of observable results), implementable (really feasible), achievable (based on constraints and resources), and timed (achievable in a given period of time)
ALICE *Nursery physician*	*For sure from tomorrow with my team I will try to give more feedback and to ask for more feedback and feedback also from my nurses, from tomorrow I will say better what they have to say on the phone in the communications and I will try to support them by listening.*		
MICHELA *Debriefer*	*Having a closed-circuit communication with your nurses: very good, thanks Alice. What did you Giulia learn from this simulation?*		
GIULIA *Neonatologist*	*I take home a reflection on the error, in the sense that from tomorrow, I will try not to underline the error of the other to point it out or judge it, but I will try to point it out to say that we all can make mistakes and we can improve together with our feedbacks.*		
MICHELA *Debriefer*	*Can you translate that into concrete action?*		
GIULIA *Neonatologist*	*Yes, I want to try this scenario with my colleagues, with a debriefing afterward, to test our group performance and to share what I learned today. Moreover, a similar situation has already happened to me: it was an urgent caesarean section for placental abruption that happened right at the time of the shift change at the beginning of the night shift. At that moment, I immediately thought to ask for help and to call the on-call service because the situation was dramatic. In fact, the baby was 33 weeks preterm, no heart rate, not breathing, and absolutely atonic, and when we started resuscitation, after a few minutes, an anesthetist suggested to stop resuscitation, but we went on; the on-call nurse arrived in the meantime, and we did everything we had to do until the end, as in this scenario we just did, and then luckily the baby recovered!*	●—▶	During the concluding phase one should not "go back" to the analysis of what happened. But in this case one of the participants is making the reflection that their own experiences that they have lived in reality are similar to those lived in the simulation scenario. The debriefer makes an exception in this case, as he/she feels that this sharing of lived experience is important and functional.

Speaker	Dialogue		Comments
MICHELA *Debriefer*	*Thank you, Giulia, for sharing with us this experience of yours, so I understand that this simulation would have been useful to you before that situation?*		
GIULIA *Neonatologist*	*Absolutely yes, there are some emergencies so difficult and not frequent that when they occur it is rare that you feel prepared; that's why I, like Sabrina, stress the importance of having tried, of having simulated.*		
DANIELA *Nurse*	*I also agree with what Giulia said, I take home the importance of the debriefing to fix the points and to reflect together; the debriefing for me is not only important after a simulation, but it would be important also during the work, after a critical situation, it should be a routine. Immediately after an emergency, we can't take that time to say "how did it go?" or "could we have done something else?", because maybe you are at the end of the shift… instead, I think it would be useful to sit down for a moment and say "ok, we did it, it went well, but maybe…." That's what I really miss about debriefing, so I'm going to try to propose it to my head nurse!*		
MICHELA *Debriefer*	*So, Daniela, if I understand you correctly, you take home the importance of debriefing, and you will try to use this method in your clinical practice. And how are you going to bring it into your daily practice?*	●—→	The debriefer brings back the concreteness of the intentions and tries to test the feasibility of what the participant has set out
DANIELA *Nurse*	*Yes, first of all I'll talk about it with my head nurse, and I'll start to do it in my own small way within my shift with the trainee nurses and why not maybe also with the doctors; I'll try to do some debriefing not only when there are situations gone wrong but also in the routine.*		

Speaker	Dialogue		Comments
MICHELA *Debriefer*	*Thank you, Daniela. That's quite a commitment! (silence)* *Well, if you have nothing else to add, before concluding, I would also like to share with you what I learned from this simulation: as a debriefer psychologist, from tomorrow, I will try to look into the eyes of my interlocutor, as we discovered together in this debriefing. For a more effective communication, it is essential to look the other person in the eyes.*	●—→	In a circular learning perspective, the debriefer also shares what he/she learned from the simulation. The SMART goal also applies to the debriefer; we cannot demand from our learners what we do not do ourselves first, so the debriefer sets the example by taking home a valuable reflection for his role and profession. He also concludes by using evocative language, speaking in images or metaphors, to leave a suggestion for the participants that functions as an anchor and emotional stabilization of the discoveries made by the participants... "change eyes, touch heart"
	Well, I sincerely thank you for your participation and effort to put yourself out there, thank you all for this interesting debriefing moment (pause for a few seconds). *As in every sport, there is need of practice and training to maintain a good level of performance, so the simulation is a gym where we can train and the important thing is that we train together. If during a football match a goal is scored, it's thanks to the whole team! Each of us can make a difference in the team.*		

Appendix B: Debriefing with Residents

Scenario Title
Postpartum hemorrhage

Participants and Roles
IVAN: debriefer
GRAZIELLA: midwife
STEFANO: nurse
SARA: obstetrician
ELEONORA: anesthesiology resident
SABRINA: anesthesiologist

Simulation Site
In the simulation center

Scenario Description
Five third-year anesthesia residents attending the obstetrics department and delivery room participate in this scenario. Learners were assigned one of the following roles prior to the scenario: obstetrician, anesthesiologist (senior), anesthesia resident, midwife, and nurse. Participants were instructed to behave and act according to their knowledge but tried to empathize with their assigned roles.

The role exchange method is one of the methods practiced in order to make participants practice living and assuming the point of view of the colleagues and/or team with whom they usually relate in their clinical activity. It is a very effective experience in didactic terms, provided that the participants have a minimum multidisciplinary technical background and have already had experience in the clinical setting in which the simulated scenario takes place.

The scenario proposes a case of postpartum hemorrhage due to uterine atony, with the patient in an initial state of hemorrhagic shock.

Debriefing

Descriptive Phase

Speaker	Dialogue		Comments
IVAN *Debriefer*	*Now we're going to proceed with the debriefing, which is structured in three phases: a first descriptive phase, in which we describe what we saw and what happened when we entered the scenario; an analytical phase in which we'll delve into the behaviors and events, examining the critical issues and whether and how we could have done things differently; and then the concluding phase, which is what we take home.* *Let's start with who entered the scenario first, which are Stefano, who was the nurse; Graziella, who was the midwife; and Sara, who was the obstetrician.* *Stefano, when you came in, what did you see?*	●—▶	If learners have entered the scenario at different times, the initial question of the descriptive phase can be asked starting with the first person who entered and then, in temporal order, to all the others. The advantage of this way of proceeding is that everyone can complete the story of the other, and the group can thus become aware that if effective communication is practiced, those who intervene when the scenario has already begun may have a very different view of the facts from those who entered first and vice versa The story of the scenario is reassembled through what each person has seen and perceived and therefore experienced. This process is highly educational as it makes the participants, still subliminally, realize that what they have experienced does not always coincide with the point of view of the other team member or leader and that there may be borderline cases in which no one or only a few had a clear idea of what it was about
STEFANO *Nurse*	*I saw blood-soaked patches, blood on the ground, the patient bleeding…*		
IVAN *Debriefer*	*Thank you, Stefano. Then what happened, Graziella?*		
GRAZIELLA *Midwife*	*The patient was very sweaty; she said she was sick, we monitored her, and we immediately realized that she was not hemodynamically stable…*		
IVAN *Debriefer*	*(Nodding) Ok*		

Speaker	Dialogue		Comments
GRAZIELLA *Midwife*	*So, I suggested to call the anesthesiologist immediately, but I was blocked by Sara, the gynecologist, who had a different opinion and took the situation in hand and started to manage that part which, according to me, was more of anesthesiological competence…*		
IVAN *Debriefer*	*All right Graziella, we'll look more closely at your comments later. You Sara (obstetrician), then you took charge of the situation, and what did you do?*	●—▶	The participant has an urgent need to comment immediately on the scenario by giving his opinion. At this stage, the debriefer should welcome this but postpone the discussion to the analytical phase, so as not to interrupt the flow of the descriptive phase, for example, "What you are telling me is too important and deserves more in-depth analysis. Write it down on a piece of paper or remember it, we will certainly talk about it in a few minutes. First, however, let's finish understanding together what happened and what you saw, so that we can establish what it was about." In all cases, the debriefer will write down the participant's observations and will find a way to talk about them again in the analytical phase, as they represent a training need of one of the participants
SARA *Obstetrician*	*We went in, and we saw many wet patches of blood, but we didn't evaluate exactly the blood loss, for example, I didn't look in the collection bag how much blood there was. We immediately monitored the patient; we saw that the blood pressure was low, and there was tachycardia, so the patient was still in compensation, and the saturation was still good. We asked for a blood sample so we could assess whether to do blood products. We increased the fluid infusion rate and added oxytocin. Then, because the patient was not improving, we called the anesthesiologist.*		

Speaker	Dialogue		Comments
IVAN *Debriefer*	*Good. So, the anesthesiologists arrived. So, let's turn to them: Eleonora, you were assigned the role of the trainee, what did you see?*		
ELEONORA *Anesthesiology Resident*	*When we arrived, the bleeding was controlled, but the patient was always unstable. Sara, the obstetrician, gave us a summary of the patient's clinical situation…*		
IVAN *Debriefer*	*All right, thank you. Sabrina, would you like to finish the story?*		
SABRINA *Anesthesiologist*	*Yes, as soon as I arrived, I noticed the blood loss in the collection bag. I asked Graziella if the uterus was hypotonic. Basically, the patient was hypotensive. When we got the analysis and I saw that she had 8.5 hemoglobin, I would have asked for blood immediately. I was afraid the patient would lose consciousness, and, I don't know if it was right, I prepared to intubate her…in case she lost consciousness….*		
IVAN *Debriefer*	*We'll investigate that later. Just keep telling the facts: what you saw and what you did.*	●→	The debriefer postpones the discussion to the following analytical phase avoiding to interrupt the flow of the descriptive phase

Speaker	Dialogue		Comments
SABRINA *Anesthesiologist*	*As soon as I arrived, I saw the patient hypotensive and tachycardic. I auscultated her, and there were no problems. I saw that oxytocin therapy had already been started, and in case the patient did not respond to therapy, I would prescribe second-line uterotonics. I prescribed additional fluids and further tests and alerted the blood bank to have plasma and blood brought in. I then saw that the patient was beginning to desaturate…and then the blood came in and the simulation ended.*		
IVAN *Debriefer*	*Thank you, Sabrina. Is there anyone who would like to add anything?*		
SARA *Obstetrician*	*We could have been neater!*		
IVAN *Debriefer*	*Yes, that's an important comment, but we'll look at that in a little bit: is there anything to add to complete the story?*	●→	Again, the debriefer welcomes the learner's input and postpones the discussion to the analytical phase
SARA *Obstetrician*	*We did plasma expanders and vasopressors, and we called for an ultrasound exam to assess the state of the uterus.*		
IVAN *Debriefer*	*Perfect. So, correct me if I'm wrong, from what you've described, this was a bleeding patient—but the cause of the bleeding is clear to everyone?*		
SARA *Obstetrician*	*A uterus that didn't contract, a uterine atony!*		
ALL	*(Nodding)*		

Speaker	Dialogue		Comments
IVAN *Debriefer*	*Was that clear to everyone? If I understood correctly, it was therefore a postpartum hemorrhage caused by an atonic uterus.*	●—▶	The debriefer's summary, with which the descriptive phase ends, can also be very brief and technical. In this case, it is the diagnosis made by the team that is restated and agreed with everyone With the debriefer's summary, both the participants and the debriefer find out whether everyone perceived the scenario in the same way and confirm that they agree with what happened
ALL	*(Nodding) Yes*		

Analytic Phase

Speaker	Dialogue		Comments
IVAN *Debriefer*	*Well if we're all clear on what this was about, let's move on. Let's proceed with the analytical phase. Let's start with you, Graziella: What's the best thing you've done as a midwife?*	●—▶	"What is the best thing you've done?" is the question that lets the learner know that they have done many good things and that they are being asked to choose the best. This is one of the most effective formulations of the first question when using the plus/delta technique. It is in fact very powerful. Starting with the positives and assuming that there have been positives, inviting the learner to report the best, usually pleasantly surprises the learner as they are usually mainly focused on seeing what went wrong or what they think they did wrong and expect criticism rather than praise. This first question sets him up well for the analytical process of debriefing. Moreover, it makes him discover how there are always positives, even unconscious, in our clinical behaviors
GRAZIELLA *Midwife*	*I followed the team leader a lot, which was Sara (obstetrician) at the beginning, and then I suggested calling the anesthetist, although she took over.*		

Speaker	Dialogue		Comments
IVAN *Debriefer*	*Yeah, all right, then what?*		
GRAZIELLA *Midwife*	*Maybe I should have helped Stefano (nurse) a little bit more...*		
IVAN *Debriefer*	*But that's not "what you've done right..."*	●→	Debriefing dialogue is a structured, guided dialogue of the debriefer in accordance with various communication techniques. If the answer is not appropriate to the question or if the participant tries to be evasive, the participant should be gently brought back to answer the question posed. In this case the participant is self-criticizing, but this is not the answer the debriefer intends to elicit with the question "What is the best thing you have done"
GRAZIELLA *Midwife*	*(Laughs embarrassed...and then silent)*		
IVAN *Debriefer*	*Is there anyone who wants to help Graziella (midwife) understand the best things she has done? You, Stefano, for example?*	●→	If the learner does not find any positive thing in what he/she did during the scenario, the others in the team will help him/her. In fact, if, as sometimes happens, the learner does not find any positive aspect, the debriefer will have to ask the same question to the other members of the team, and usually there is always someone who has noticed positive attitudes of someone else. If the group can't find any positive behavior either, the debriefer, before reporting what he/she has noticed, can resort to an explanatory video sequence, which will give the answer that will certainly be much more powerful and effective than any statement he/she made
STEFANO *Nurse*	*Graziella (midwife) was a good member of the team, she did very well what was required of her...*		

Speaker	Dialogue		Comments
IVAN *Debriefer*	*Thank you, Stefano. What about you Sara (obstetrician), what do you think? Is there anything else that you noticed that Graziella (midwife) got right?*		
SARA *Obstetrician*	*Yes, there was a very good closed-circuit communication between me and Graziella!*		
IVAN *Debriefer*	*Could you give me an example, please?*		
SARA *Obstetrician*	*Whenever I asked her to do something, such as administer a medication or measure blood pressure, she would give me immediate feedback. I felt comfortable with this.*		
IVAN *Debriefer*	*See, Graziella, how many things your teammates have noticed? Closed loop communication is very important!*	●──▶	The debriefer achieved his aim. Graziella's (midwife) positive behaviors were noticed and made explicit by the team and not by the debriefer. The recognition by the teammates acts as a positive reinforcement on the actions performed by Graziella, who comes out not only gratified (she smiles and nods) but certainly strengthened in her virtuous behaviors. The debriefer himself emphasizes, at this point, the positivity of the participant's virtuous behavior and can do so because both the team and the participant themselves have recognized it. In practice, the debriefer puts into practice Descartes' phrase: "No one can understand anything well and make it his own when he has learned it from another, as opposed to when he has learned it himself"
GRAZIELLA *Midwife*	*(Nods and smiles with satisfaction)*		
IVAN *Debriefer*	*And you, Sara, what's the best thing you've done?*		

Speaker	Dialogue		Comments
SARA *Obstetrician*	*I think I was good in the handover when the anesthesiologist arrived, I also think I took a step backward passing the leadership to her, but then I kept re-evaluating the patient, always thinking inside myself what would have been the next step to take.*		
IVAN *Debriefer*	*Thank you, Sara. Good. And is there anything you would have done differently?*		
SARA *Obstetrician*	*With hindsight, maybe we hesitated too much on the issue of uterotonics; we should have been more insistent.*		
IVAN *Debriefer*	*Okay, so you specifically what would you have done differently?*	●—▶	Note that whenever the participant's answer is not specific enough or is even partly evasive, the debriefer rephrases the question in order to facilitate further investigation
SARA *Obstetrician*	*I would have increased the dose of oxytocin much earlier, and I would have used prostaglandins earlier.*		
IVAN *Debriefer*	*(Nodding) Ok*		
SARA *Obstetrician*	*Basically, I would have been more aggressive…*		
IVAN *Debriefer*	*Thank you, Sara. And you, Stefano: What's the best thing you've done?*		

Speaker	Dialogue		Comments
STEFANO *Nurse*	*I felt projected into my role as a nurse; I felt different from the reality that I live every day as a resident anesthesiologist, and maybe I felt a little bit free from responsibilities. The best thing I did was to provide telephone communication. I did what was asked of me in a precise and timely manner. The artery was in situ, but I didn't understand if I should cannulate it or not, but then eventually I did the blood gas analysis from the arterial access that I found. There was a venous extension that didn't work, and I changed it, etc. I did what a nurse does, trying to be as realistic as possible to empathize....*		
IVAN *Debriefer*	*I'm very interested in what you said about "disempowerment." Can you elaborate on that please?*	●→	The debriefer takes advantage of Stefano's experience as a nurse to investigate the positivity of the role exchange method. He could have explored the topic in more depth with the rest of the team, but in this case, he decided not to go into it to avoid the interruption of the conversation flow with a new topic that would have taken the discussion far. Alternatively, he could have suspended the reflection on "what it feels like to put yourself in the shoes of another professional" and then come back to the topic later
STEFANO *Nurse*	*I wanted to say that since in the real life I'm a specialist in anesthesia, as a doctor, I'm used to feeling the weight of decision-making responsibility, and today, in the scenario, when I played the role of nurse, I didn't have this problem, but I focused my attention on what they ordered me to do...*		

Speaker	Dialogue		Comments
IVAN *Debriefer*	*And was this a positive or negative experience?*		
STEFANO *Nurse*	*Absolutely positive! I was able to put myself in the shoes of another professional figure, and I think I will take this into account the next time I find myself in a similar situation in real life.*		
IVAN *Debriefer*	*I got it. Thanks Stefano! You Eleonora?*		
ELEONORA *Anesthesiology Resident*	*I put myself in the shoes of a resident, which is easy, because I am also in reality, who observes, scrutinizes, and tries to learn, because it was the first time, she saw a postpartum hemorrhage. The thing I did best I think was to have observed the situation and my tutor, with the spirit of "I observe, I memorize, and I learn." However, in this way, I think I participated very little from a clinical perspective....*		
IVAN *Debriefer*	*Is there anything you would have done differently?*		
ELEONORA *Anesthesiology Resident*	*I missed a little bit the communication with Sabrina, who was the senior anesthesiologist...*		
SABRINA *Anesthesiologist*	*(Nodding and agreeing)*		
ELEONORA *Anesthesiology Resident*	*Yes, communicating together with questions like: what would you do... I don't know...*		
IVAN *Debriefer*	*Give me an example, please.*	●⟶	Asking for a concrete example helps the participant better explain his thoughts and his fellow students to better understand and identify with the situation being described
ELEONORA *Anesthesiology Resident*	*To establish a common program that would tell me what I could be useful in, for example*		
IVAN *Debriefer*	*And so, what have you done?*	●⟶	Being the learner's answer evasive, the debriefer reformulates the question in order to facilitate further investigation

Speaker	Dialogue		Comments
ELEONORA *Anesthesiology Resident*	*I would have liked to ask, for example, which was the plan B inside which I would have inserted myself…*		
IVAN *Debriefer*	*And how do you think you could have done to improve communication with your tutor? If you had a time machine, and you could go back and repeat the scenario, what would you do?*		
ELEONORA *Anesthesiology Resident*	*Talk much more to the tutor, very simply!*		
IVAN *Debriefer*	*And why did you fail to do so in this case: did you not want to "waste time" or were you afraid of a judgement on your skills/competencies?*	●——▶	Each discovery by the learner is followed by a debriefer request for further investigation. The question is "Why." In this case, an illusion of alternatives question is used
ELEONORA *Anesthesiology Resident*	*Perhaps because in a moment of panic in which I saw you having to make important decisions, I didn't interfere in order not to make you lose time. Maybe I was in her way.*		
IVAN *Debriefer*	*So, if I understand you correctly, correct me if I'm wrong, you thought you were wasting the time of your mentor who was making decisions. Let's hear from her: do you, Sabrina, think you would have wasted time if you had confronted your resident?*	●——▶	The debriefer rephrases using participant's own words to facilitate the participant's awareness process of what happened. It is often good, after rephrasing, to ask for confirmation from all team members

Speaker	Dialogue		Comments
SABRINA *Anesthesiologist*	*No, absolutely not. It's true that as soon as I arrived, I was thinking about the clinical situation of the patient, but I gave to my resident the tasks, for example, to prepare the medicines, to prepare the airway aids, so that if the clinical situation had degenerated quickly, we would have had everything ready. I counted on her, and from that point of view I was calm because I knew there was someone I could trust. But thinking about it, maybe, I never asked for feedback. For example, I asked the obstetrician if the uterus was tonic but I didn't wait or evaluate his answer...*		
IVAN *Debriefer*	*Considering what you said, then what would you have done differently to improve communication with your resident? Do you think it might have been helpful to have better communication with her?*		
SABRINA *Anesthesiologist*	*Maybe I should have given you some tasks without waiting for you to propose...*		
IVAN *Debriefer*	*And this would have been useful?*		
SABRINA *Anesthesiologist*	*(Laughs embarrassed)*		
SARA *Obstetrician*	*It happens to me in real life all the time! Tutors don't communicate with residents.*		
ELEONORA *Anesthesiology Resident*	*It happens to me too, often the tutors ignore us...*		
IVAN *Debriefer*	*This is very interesting: in everyday life, what could you do to avoid or better or improve these behaviors? Do you think that good communication between a leader and the trainee is important? For example, what would you Eleonora have done differently in order to get Sabrina's attention?*	●──▶	The participants are comparing the simulation scenario experience with his real life. The debriefer does not miss the opportunity to analyze in depth the topic

Speaker	Dialogue		Comments
ELEONORA *Anesthesiology Resident*	*Perhaps in such a concise moment, it was not opportune*		
SABRINA *Anesthesiologist*	*Honestly, the fact that I wasn't disturbed in the decision-making moment when the moment was critical made it easier for me. I appreciated the fact that my resident took a step back...*		
IVAN *Debriefer*	*In this case, it wasn't the most useful thing for you, and so it was the right thing to do at that particular time....*		
ELEONORA *Anesthesiology Resident*	*Yes, but maybe afterward, when the tension had subsided, we could have done a briefing together: she would have explained me what was happening, and I would have understood and cooperated with more awareness.*		
SABRINA *Anesthesiologist*	*Yes, and I think it's the right thing to do, and we didn't do it, because we were in a hurry, and maybe we were anxious to intervene on the patient.*		
IVAN *Debriefer*	*And how would you go about doing that in these cases to communicate even in a time of emergency?*		
SABRINA *Anesthesiologist*	*Stop for a moment and reflect on the situation!... Yes, we should have stopped and communicated!*		
ELEONORA *Anesthesiology Resident*	*Yes, perhaps that would have been the best strategy, I agree.*		
IVAN *Debriefer*	*Do you know of any strategies suggested by CRM in this regard?*	●—▶	The learners have made an educational discovery, and the debriefer re-proposes it by recalling CRM guidelines
SABRINA *Anesthesiologist* and ELEONORA *Anesthesiology Resident*	*(Together) Of course! The 10x10 rule! Stopping to check in together!*		
IVAN *Debriefer*	*Do we all agreed?*		
ALL	*(Nodding)*		

Speaker	Dialogue		Comments
IVAN *Debriefer*	*Is it, then, better to let confusion take over or to communicate in a structured way?*	●→	The illusion of alternatives question consolidates the participants' discovery
ALL	*Obviously the second one!*		
IVAN *Debriefer*	*Stopping to gain time: indiscriminate doing without stopping does not always produce efficiency! (silence). It's a bit like leaving later to arrive earlier! (silence)*	●→	The previous type of question is now followed by a catchphrase and a silent pause to produce an "echo effect" and reinforce the group's discovery
	But let's not forget Sabrina; now I'm going to ask you, too: what's the best thing you think you've done?	●→	The debriefer deliberately reminds everyone aloud that one of the participants did not have the opportunity to contribute to the reflective conversation ("but let's not forget Sabrina"). In this way, he shows everyone how the contribution of each participants is important for the learning of all
SABRINA *Anesthesiologist*	*I don't know, what did I do right? I really don't know.*		
IVAN *Debriefer*	*Is there anyone who can help her?*	●→	Since the learner does not find any positive action she did during the scenario, the debriefer asks the same question to the other team members. Normally someone has noticed positive attitudes of someone else
ELEONORA *Anesthesiology Resident*	*The fact that she provided a plan B*		
STEFANO *Nurse*	*She re-evaluated the patient several times.*		
IVAN *Debriefer*	*Did you see that? You've done at least two very important things, by the way, all suggested by the CRM as well! Is there anything you would have done differently?*		
SABRINA *Anesthesiologist*	*I would have asked more information to the obstetrician who talked to me but I didn't really listen to her...*		
IVAN *Debriefer*	*So, what would you do now?*		

Speaker	Dialogue		Comments
SABRINA *Anesthesiologist*	*Instead of rushing the patient, I would stop and listen to what the obstetrician has to say, have a briefing with her, and go over the history and clinical data together.*		
IVAN *Debriefer*	*So, if I understand you correctly, correct me if I'm wrong, you wouldn't go straight to the patient, but you would first engage with the team in the room to understand the clinical situation...*	●→	The same words in different sequences produce different results. This statement by Pascal fits well with the methodology of the restructuring paraphrase. The debriefer uses this technique to define a problem with each of the learners after asking open-ended questions. After a sequence of two or three questions, the debriefer provides the learner with a redefinition of his findings to check his understanding and to send him back a reformulated version of what was said, thus facilitating the process of change
SABRINA *Anesthesiologist*	*Yes, exactly. And also, I would have distributed better the roles and the workload of the team. In this way we would have worked with more order and efficiency, because I saw so much confusion.*		
IVAN *Debriefer*	*And in practice what would you do?*		
SABRINA *Anesthesiologist*	*I would impose myself a little bit more, assigning to each one a task. In fact, I was not the leader of the group.*		
IVAN *Debriefer*	*But I'll ask Sara this: was there a leader?*		
SARA *Obstetrician*	*I gave Sabrina space, I feel like I shared leadership with her.*		
IVAN *Debriefer*	*Was there a specific leader?*		
SARA *Obstetrician*	*In my opinion it's definitely Sabrina, the senior anesthetist, who was the leader of the group!*		

Speaker	Dialogue		Comments
IVAN *Debriefer*	*You, Graziella, who were the midwife, who did you feel as a leader?*	●→	When it is not entirely clear whether there has been leadership or who the leader has been, it can be very helpful to hear from the team. In this case, the debriefer asks to the midwife and nurse, who are in a privileged position to observe the behaviors of physician leaders
GRAZIELLA *Midwife*	*In the first part of the scenario, before the arrival of the anesthetists, the leader was the obstetrician (Sara), and then, the leadership was taken by the senior anesthetist (Sabrina).*		
IVAN *Debriefer*	*What did you see that from? What did Sabrina, who was the senior anesthesiologist, did or said, and what made you think that she had become the leader?*	●→	The debriefer is not satisfied with the statement "Sabrina has been a leader" but delves deeper by asking "what behaviors did you get that from?", facilitating the process of recognizing leadership from behaviors. His aim is that the entire group acquire and/or remember which behaviors distinguish leadership
GRAZIELLA *Midwife*	*She was the one who decided the therapies and told us what we had to do.*		
IVAN *Debriefer*	*So, if I understand you correctly, correct me if I'm wrong, you saw a handoff between leaders because Sabrina since she entered the scenario has been making the most important decisions and organizing the work of the team by distributing the workloads. And these are some of the behaviors, as we all know, that characterize a leader, correct?*		
GRAZIELLA *Midwife*	*Yes, exactly.*		
IVAN *Debriefer*	*What do you think, Stefano?*		
STEFANO *Nurse*	*For me, the leadership was a bit confused.*		
IVAN *Debriefer*	*Why? Can you elaborate on that point?*		

Speaker	Dialogue		Comments
STEFANO *Nurse*	*I don't know, I had the feeling of not having a reference figure. I received instructions from both the obstetrician and the anesthetist, and I couldn't distinguish the reference leader between the two.*		
IVAN *Debriefer*	*And how do you think the two co-leaders could have done to be clearer?*		
STEFANO *Nurse*	*In my opinion, we should have had a briefing together, and they should not have excluded us. If I had been involved as a nurse in their decision-making discussions maybe I would have had less confusion.*		
IVAN *Debriefer*	*And so if you had been the leader, what would you have done differently to make this leadership transition clearer for everyone? What would you have done to make sure that your team didn't experience the feelings of uncertainty that you did?*	●→	Asking those who played the role of nurses what they would have done if they had been the leader has a double value, both for them and for the leaders, who in this way does not feel directly involved and therefore directly judged for their work
STEFANO *Nurse*	*If I had been one of the two leaders, I would have stopped and checked the situation with the whole team and not just with my co-leader. In this way I would have involved everyone!*		
IVAN *Debriefer*	*And you who have been leaders, what do you think? Do you agree?*		
SARA *Obstetrician*	*Yes, maybe we should have stopped the team and made the program together; at that point, our collaborators would have realized better that I was handing over to whoever had more competences than me, that is to say the anesthesiologist.*		

Speaker	Dialogue		Comments
IVAN *Debriefer*	*You all agree?*		
ALL	*(Nodding) Yes.*		
IVAN *Debriefer*	*So if I understand you correctly, correct me if I'm wrong, stopping the team and discussing the case involving the whole team instead of just discussing it between co-leaders makes everyone gain situational awareness, and everyone works better: is that what you meant?*	●—▶	The debriefer provides all learners with a redefinition of the information gathered and to send back to them a reframed version of what has been said—thus facilitating the change process. He then verifies the understanding (the diagnostic hypothesis)
ALL	*(Nodding) Yes*		

Application Phase

Speaker	Dialogue		Comments
IVAN *Debriefer*	*We now move on to the concluding or application phase, during which each of us will share what we learned from this scenario. Sabrina (anesthesiologist) what are you taking home? Tomorrow, you go back to your hospital, and maybe you will be in a similar situation. Is there anything you will do differently from what you used to do before this simulation scenario?*	●—▶	
SABRINA *Anesthesiologist*	*I take home the importance of planning and being prepared to the precipitation of the clinical situation. I didn't feel anxious in this situation, and I'm satisfied because what we had to do we did it…*		

Speaker	Dialogue		Comments
IVAN *Debriefer*	*Yes, but specifically what is it that you're taking home?*	●—→	In order to make application phase effective for everyone, the debriefer asks each participant what they take home and how this can become a small, but sure, agent of change, necessary for what was learned in the debriefing Being the proposed take-home too general, the debriefer keeps questioning more specifically. He wants to achieve the identification of a SMART goal, thus the smallest step to a truly actionable change which depends solely on the learner (*you can't change things that don't depend on us*). The debriefer invites participants to use "performative" language, such as "I propose that in the next emergency situation I will do...." In this case the utterance of the word is itself the performance of an action that creates, in fact, a new reality, and not simply the saying of something
SABRINA *Anesthesiologist*	*The fact that I have to learn to be tidier and take care of the work organization when I have the leadership that, in my opinion, I missed a bit in this scenario.*		
IVAN *Debriefer*	*Trying to be a "tidier" leader. Thank you, Sabrina. What about you Sara, what are you taking home?*		

Speaker	Dialogue		Comments
SARA *Obstetrician*	*I am obsessed with protocols because I think that when I become a specialist I will have to manage the clinic according to protocols. But if we are here it's to learn: being a leader is difficult, and the first thing to do is to train yourself to distribute workloads well within the team, because that's what makes the difference. You may know how to apply clinical protocols perfectly, but if you don't have a collaborative team, things don't work.*		
IVAN *Debriefer*	*So what, Sara?*		
SARA *Obstetrician*	*When I happen to be a leader, the first thing I will do is assign tasks to each of my team members.*		
IVAN *Debriefer*	*Assign clear tasks to everyone. Good! Thank you, Sara! Graziella, what are you taking home?*	●─▶	After each of the participants has identified a personal SMART goal to take home, the debriefer summarizes it using the redefinition technique. This paraphrase also serves to reinforce the findings, highlighting how they came from below and not imposed a priori by the debriefer, confirming his role as "facilitator" and not "teacher." The debriefer concludes always thanking the participant
GRAZIELLA *Midwife*	*I, from what I learned from this scenario, would say that I take home the communication with my colleagues because, in my opinion, I was a bit lacking. I noticed that I often put myself aside when I would have been more helpful if I had proposed myself.*		
IVAN *Debriefer*	*(Nodding)* *And so specifically, what do you plan to do during the next emergency that comes your way?*		

Speaker	Dialogue		Comments
GRAZIELLA *Midwife*	*I'll be careful to propose myself even if the leader neglects me, because I've understood that a good team member must not only collaborate but can also propose himself...*		
IVAN *Debriefer*	*Propose yourself. Of course, every leader needs each of the team members; they can't see everything, and proposing yourself is certainly the best way to help them. OK, thanks! And you Stefano?*		
STEFANO *Nurse*	*Like Graziella, I take home the importance of good communication between all participants.*		
IVAN *Debriefer*	*And specifically, personally? You're going back to the hospital tomorrow and what do you change?*	●→	The debriefer asks to define a SMART goal, which more likely leads the learner to effective change being dependent on him, feasible, measurable, timed, and emotionally internalized
STEFANO *Nurse*	*So, since it gave me peace of mind to have within the simulation, a well-organized hospital, I take home the anticipation and planning: the next time an emergency happens to me, I will pay attention to who is there, who to trust, and who to call for help and know the resources I have available ...*		
IVAN *Debriefer*	*Anticipating problems, then. Thank you, Stefano! And you, Eleonora?*		
ELEONORA *Anesthesiology Resident*	*I too take home the improvement in communication and also the idea of being able to do simulations to gain more confidence that allows you to fit better into the team and therefore to collaborate better on the clinical case.*		
IVAN *Debriefer*	*And doing simulations is entirely up to you?*	●→	To be SMART, the goal has to be totally dependent on the learner. The debriefer challenges her to identify something actually feasible

Speaker	Dialogue		Comments
ELEONORA *Anesthesiology Resident*	*(Smiling) Attending courses or training sessions yes, but organizing them… just no!*		
IVAN *Debriefer*	*So, is there anything that you could do as a resident, and that's entirely up to you, and therefore is definitely and immediately achievable, to gain more confidence, improve communication, and collaborate better with the team?*	●→	The debriefer shares with the learner the key characteristics of a goal to be SMART to facilitate its identification by the learner
ELEONORA *Anesthesiology Resident*	*I propose to talk about it with my tutor and demand from him a briefing before and after every clinical case we face together!*		
IVAN *Debriefer*	*Sure! You can certainly do that! And it's a very concrete and attainable thing. Thank you, Eleonora!* *I noticed that even if not all of you knew the environment well, both the simulation room and the delivery room, you all managed to bring a result home: the patient was improving and you stabilized her. So, I personally take home the observation that sometimes you can get a result even without knowing everything if there is a proper teamwork and helping each other. You made up for your inexperience in the field with common sense, enthusiasm, and cooperation, and this can also happen in reality.* *Normally, and rightly so, we believe that following guidelines protects us from mistakes and always guarantees success. However, with simulation, we learn that almost always "knowing" or "knowing how to do" is not enough but that also good cooperation and communication in the team can significantly affect our behaviors and clinical knowledge.* *(Silent pause)* *Thank you all for this mutual learning experience!*	●→	After all participants in the session have participated in the application phase and stated what they have learned and the resulting SMART personal goal, the debriefer closes by sharing what he learned from the session, to highlight that learning in simulation is circular and benefits everyone. He ends the debriefing thanking everyone and, using an evocative language, leaving a suggestion, using a short sentence (aphorism, story, anecdote, quotation) that works as an anchor and emotional stabilization of the discovery made by participants (echo effect)

Appendix C: Debriefing with Regular Staff After In Situ Simulation

Scenario Title
The flooding storm
Iatrogenic rupture of pulmonary artery with sudden bleeding and subsequent cardiac arrest

Participants and Roles
LEONARDO: debriefer
BEATRICE: young anesthesiologist
ALESSANDRA: anesthesia nurse
ARIANNA: thoracic surgeon
MARK: assistant surgeon
SOFIA: scrub nurse
MARY: OR nurse

Simulation Site
In situ (on site, in the OR)

Scenario Description
This is an in situ simulation. The scenario takes place in the cardiothoracic operating room and starts with the patient under general anesthesia on the operating table in the appropriate position for elective left thoracoscopic lobectomy. The surgeon accidentally injures the pulmonary artery with rapid bleeding that requires thoracotomy and immediate clamping of the vessel. Massive bleeding involves hemorrhagic shock with bradycardia up to the cardiac arrest. The team is activated for an open chest cardiac massage and a volume replacement (with possible blood recovery). The resolution of the cardiac arrest and the return to spontaneous circulation (ROSC) occurs only after defibrillation with internal plaques. The scenario included two surgical solutions, pneumonectomy or the activation of the ECMO Mobile team.

The participants are healthcare professionals from the hospital and play the same professional role in the scenario as they do in life.

Debriefing

De-roling
Immediately after finishing the scenario, as they leave the surgical unit, the debriefer invites the participants to take off the surgical gowns and facilitates the de-roling in the room nearby, trying to get the scenario participants to express their emotions.

Speaker	Dialogue		Comments
LEONARDO *Debriefer*	*Thank you for participating in this training session.* *Before moving to the debriefing room, I'd like to invite you to share your emotions and how you feel right now. Let's go around. Who would like to start?*	●──▶	The debriefer encourages the learners to decompress and step out of the role they played during the scenario. In addition, he wants to understand the emotional state of each participant
Beatrice *Young* *anesthesiologist*	*(After a few seconds, she raises her hand and looks at all the participants almost asking the permission to start)* *May I start?*		
LEONARDO *Debriefer*	*Please, Beatrice. Go ahead.*		.
Beatrice *Young* *anesthesiologist*	*I think it went well. We recognized the emergency situation immediately, we started the emergency procedures, and we communicated easily, what else?* *We resuscitated the patient when he suffered the VF. We were a good team, since we all knew each other already. I was fine. I feel comfortable.*		
LEONARDO *Debriefer*	*Thanks, Beatrice, for your comments. We'll go back into the details of what you generally described in a short while. Right now, just focus on your emotions, such as happiness, fear, sadness, or anger. Which emotion did you predominantly feel?*	●──▶	The answer was not consistent with the question. The majority of people often start with a generic evaluation of performance and a short description of actions and facts. The debriefer asks again to investigate the perceived emotion and proposes the basic emotions to facilitate the sharing
Beatrice *Young* *anesthesiologist*	*Well, I think I'm happy. As I said we managed the case well, as a good group.*		
LEONARDO *Debriefer*	*Thank you, Beatrice. What about you, Alessandra?*	●──▶	Now the debriefer addresses the question directly to a learner to give the sense of going around
ALESSANDRA *anesthesia nurse*	*I'm satisfied. But at the beginning, I was a little bit anxious.*		
LEONARDO *Debriefer*	*Satisfaction and anxiety. Thank you, Alessandra.* *Sofia? What about you? How are you feeling?*		

Speaker	Dialogue		Comments
SOFIA *Scrub nurse*	*I had some anxiety too. The scenario was very realistic.*		
LEONARDO *Debriefer*	*Thank you for sharing, Sofia. Arianna, how do you feel?*		
ARIANNA *Thoracic surgeon*	*I was calm. I had the situation under control. A great team with me. So, probably happiness is the most appropriate emotion I feel.*		
LEONARDO *Debriefer*	*OK, thanks. And you Mark? It's your turn now.*		
MARK *Assistant surgeon*	*A lot of adrenaline. Fortunately, I observed that Arianna had everything under control, and this helped me keep calm. But probably, if I have to say the predominant emotion, I guess fear is the right one.*		
LEONARDO *Debriefer*	*And you Mary?*		
MARY *OR nurse*	*I was excited. I had a lot of thinking to do. Everyone was demanding. I felt a little bit overwhelmed in a given moment. But I am satisfied with the way the team dealt with the difficulties. Yes, satisfaction is my main feeling, I'd say.*		
LEONARDO *Debriefer*	*Thanks, all. It's not easy to express our emotions in public. So, I really thank you. If I can wrap up, please correct me if I am wrong, you all experience good emotions due to the fact that the emergency was apparently under control and well managed; nevertheless, a few of you felt anxiety and fear.*	●→	The debriefer summarizes what everyone has experienced. He achieved his aim: he wanted everyone to verbalize the deep emotion felt during the scenario This will help motivate learners to meet their learning needs
	Now, we kindly move to the debriefing room, and we'll reflect together about what we have just experienced.		

Introduction

Speaker	Dialogue		Comments
LEONARDO *Debriefer*	*Thank you for your active participation in this training session.* *Now we'll reflect together about the actions which were taken. This is not about criticizing anyone, but, simply about improving the group's performance and also the system resilience.* *We'll proceed in this way: we'll describe what happened, and we'll analyze together what was done, paying attention to what could be improved for the patient's safety, of course, and, I'd say also ours, and finally we'll conclude sharing what we have learned from this experience and what we'll do next time in a similar, real situation. Everyone will report his or her thoughts which we will all listen to respectfully. Please avoid talking at the same time; we'll speak one at a time. I'll try to moderate and facilitate this conversation. This will be my role. We'll synthesize what emerges from this discussion into a short report for the Safety and Quality Improvement Office. There will be no judgment, criticism, or blame, but simply, I think you agree with me, we would like to identify latent threats that must be addressed and worked out.*	●—▶	The debriefer recognizes that everyone has attempted to throw themselves fully into the scenario and thanks everyone for this key effort. He also describes the structure of the following discussion and highlights the need to respect everyone's thoughts. He also reminds the learners of the rules of the session and clearly states what the purpose of the debriefing and ultimately of the whole training session

Descriptive Phase

Speaker	Dialogue		Comments
LEONARDO *Debriefer*	*Well, let's start with Arianna: what did you see, and what did you do?*	●—▶	The debriefer wants to review the case and make evident how the participants experienced it. The aim here is to check each participant's understanding of what happened in the scenario

Speaker	Dialogue		Comments
ARIANNA *Thoracic surgeon*	*We had a 65-year-old patient under general anesthesia undertaking an elective thoracoscopic lobectomy. The vital parameters and ventilators were normal, and the surgery was in progress. Suddenly, we observed an important bleeding in our operating field, very likely due to an accidental cut of a vessel. We immediately alerted Sofia to prepare the bleeding kit. We probably delayed a bit in calling Sabrina and Alessandra and to share what was happening. Our main priority was to find the vessel which was bleeding and immediately to clamp it. It's a matter of minutes before the patient dies. But yes, reflecting calmly now, I probably made a mistake: I should have alerted Sabrina sooner.*		
LEONARDO *Debriefer*	*Thanks Arianna, we'll go into these details later, don't worry. Let's keep describing what happened. Mark, do you want to continue telling us what you and Arianna did?*	●—▶	The debriefer stops Arianna since she was starting to analyze the facts. This would interrupt the flow of description and could create confusion in the participants. It's better to follow a structure. The debriefer takes note of the Arianna's comment: it must be explored in the analytic phase
MARK *Assistant surgeon*	*The bleeding was massive. I was really scared, but fortunately, Arianna found the source of the hemorrhage and was able to clamp at the second attempt. I looked up, I saw Alessandra, and I asked her about the patient's condition, and I said aloud that the patient was bleeding.*		
(LEONARDO) (Debriefer)	*Ah, ok. Alessandra, what then?*		

Speaker	Dialogue		Comments
ALESSANDRA *anesthesia nurse*	*I noticed immediately that something was wrong, and I called Sabrina who was filling in the patient chart.* *We realized that the situation was serious: the patient became unstable, the pressure went down suddenly, and the HR slowed down. The patient was shocking.* *I was asked to call the blood bank for blood products and to prepare the prohemostatic drug.*		
LEONARDO *Debriefer*	*Ok. And you Sabrina, what did you do?*		
BEATRICE *Young anesthesiologist*	*As Alessandra said, we realized that the situation was serious, we saw how much blood the aspiration device was recollecting? Since I'm not used to this type of emergency, I wanted to call the senior anesthetist. At the same time, when Arianna and Mark confirmed the massive hemorrhage, I had in mind the massive hemorrhage protocol we recently agreed upon in the hospital. So, I thought transfusion was urgent; I asked for large volumes of fluids, and I ordered for the prohemostatic drug to be brought. At the same time, I called Mary and ordered her to bring the Cell Saver. I kept looking at the monitor, and I noticed the bradycardia. I didn't have time to give the inotrope when it became a VF. I checked the pulse, and the patient was in cardiac arrest. I immediately asked Arianna to start the open chest cardiac massage, and I asked for the defibrillator with internal plaques. Only after the first shock the heart started to beat again, and we checked for the spontaneous circulation. Then the scenario was stopped.*		
LEONARDO *Debriefer*	*Thank you, Beatrice, for your report. Mary, would you like to add what you saw and what you did?*		
MARY *OR nurse*	*Actually, I was running all the time. For the defibrillator, the Cell Saver, the call. As I said earlier I felt overwhelmed. I had some trouble with the Cell Saver, I never prepared it.* *I was also called out of the OR by the ancillary who brought the blood.*		

Speaker	Dialogue		Comments
BEATRICE *Young anesthesiologist*	*Ah, I thought the blood never arrived.*		
MARY *OR nurse*	*I said clearly and aloud that the blood had arrived, and I placed the blood bags in the tray behind you.*		
LEONARDO *Debriefer*	*That's interesting. We'll discuss about it in the analytic phase of this debriefing. [a]* *Let me summarize. We all agree that this was a case of rapid massive hemorrhage in a patient under thoracoscopic lobectomy due to an accidental injury to the pulmonary artery. This led to hemorrhagic shock, to cardiac arrest as VF, and the ROSC occurred after adequate volume filling and the first shock. The scenario ended when Arianna ordered the activation of the referral ECMO mobile team. Is that correct? [b]*	●━━▶	[a] The debriefer again notices another element that must be discussed in the following phase. He addresses the importance of this element, and he reassures everyone that there will be time to delve into it [b] The debriefer synthetically reformulates the participants' experiences. The aim is to establish the starting point for the analytical phase. The debriefer also become aware of some elements in need of deeper analysis
ALL	*(All nodded and confirmed)*		

Analytic Phase

Speaker	Dialogue		Comments
LEONARDO *Debriefer*	*OK, I'd like to talk now more in deep about the actions which were taken and explore all the points of view.* *What's the best thing you did in the in the scenario that has just ended?*	●━━▶	In the analytical phase, the debriefer wants to explore and deepen the reasons for the individual and team behaviors. He starts generically asking a very open question to the team
MARK *Assistant surgeon*	*We were able to clamp the artery very soon. Otherwise, the patient would have very likely died.*		
ARIANNA *Thoracic surgeon*	*Yes, that's certainly true. But we probably delayed in alerting the anesthesiology team.*		

Speaker	Dialogue		Comments
LEONARDO *Debriefer*	*That's interesting, Arianna, you already shared this comment earlier, and I thank you for having raised it again. It was in my mind too. What was in your mind at that time?*	●→	The debriefer makes a note about Arianna's comment in the descriptive phase. He knows Arianna is feeling the need to talk about it. And the fact that Arianna shares it once again is the confirmation
ARIANNA *Thoracic surgeon*	*Of course, my priority was to find the source of bleeding and to stop it, because we all know that the time is very short and the consequences could be very bad. By the way, the anesthesiologist must be immediately made aware about of the emergency situation, so she can sustain the vital conditions and she can give us more time to find the lesion.*		
LEONARDO *Debriefer*	*Ok, correct me, please, if I'm wrong. You are saying that a sort of an early warning to the anesthesia team, but probably to the entire team would help in such a situation? What do the others think? Mary, for example, what do you think?*	●→	The debriefer is using a paraphrase to verify his understanding and to re-punctuate the sequence of events. After this, he addresses the question to Mary to avoid that the conversation being dominated by the physicians and to hint to everyone that everybody's thoughts matter
MARY *OR nurse*	*I agree. I'm in the OR, of course, but I don't see what's going on during the surgery, I mean, on the operating table. I realized it was an emergency when I heard Beatrice raise her voice to talk with Alessandra and define the to-dos with her. And at the same time, I received orders from everyone. I was neither aware they were targeting me nor what to do first.*		
LEONARDO *Debriefer*	*Thanks, Mary. One thing at a time. I guess we all agree that an immediate warning to all the team would benefit the emergency management.*		
ALL	*(Nodding)*		

Speaker	Dialogue		Comments
LEONARDO *Debriefer*	*But Mary introduced another important element. Let me understand. Are we saying that calling people by name helps activate them and makes us sure that the message has been received, or is shouting orders to everyone in the air sufficient?*	●——▶	The debriefer asks an alternative illusion question, to emphasize the importance of nonverbal communication
ARIANNA *Thoracic surgeon*	*Certainly, when we address the order, or any communication to someone specific and we grab his attention by calling him directly.*		
MARY *OR nurse*	*Actually, I realize now that I made a similar mistake when I brought the blood bags into the OR. I said I was putting them in the tray, but I didn't address my communication to Beatrice or Alessandra. They were probably too busy in doing their staff, and they were not paying attention to me.*		
ALESSANDRA *anesthesia nurse*	*Ops, In fact, I was convinced that the blood never arrived.*		
BEATRICE *Young anesthesiologist*	*Actually, I asked for the bags several times. I got that the bags had been ordered from the blood bank as protocol and they were on their way.*		
LEONARDO *Debriefer*	*Then, if I understand correctly, but, please correct me, you are telling me that in such a high-risk environment, and in addition, since we deal with time-sensitive situations, effective communication, which includes explicit messages addressed to a specific person by* name, *and I'd add closed loop, is a requirement for safe patient care delivery and an important element of teamwork.*	●——▶	After hearing the favorable opinions from the group, the debriefer uses the instrument of reframing and paraphrase to confirm the discovery made by the group (debriefer and learners) and to reinforce its effect
ALL	*(Nodding and reflecting)*		

Speaker	Dialogue		Comments
LEONARDO *Debriefer*	*Well, is there anything you would do differently next time you face a similar scenario or a similar real case? Alessandra, what do you think?*	•——►	The debriefer is satisfied with the agreement achieved about the communication effectiveness. He is confident that this will inspire some take-home messages in the following debriefing phase. He wants now to move the conversation forward and change topic. He then poses an open question, but he decides to address it to Alessandra because she hasn't spoken very much
ALESSANDRA *Anesthesia nurse*	*Well, probably, I'll check how to prepare prohemostatic drugs. I've never done it before, and it was difficult to read and follow the instructions for the first time ever.*		
LEONARDO *Debriefer*	*What do you mean exactly?*		
ALESSANDRA *Anesthesia nurse*	*Some of these drugs have a specific preparation technique and diluting process. I was not familiar with them, and it took a lot of time to stay calm and concentrate on doing the preparation. Being very expensive, the method of preparation has never been demonstrated.*		
SOFIA *Scrub nurse*	*This is very dangerous, I think. How can we pretend to be efficient and rapid if we cannot gain specific experience?*		
MARY *OR nurse*	*I had the same problem with the Cell Saver. I've never assembled all the pieces. We actually used it in another simulation, but we simply brought the device in the OR, and we pretended it was ready to use.*		
MARK *Assistant surgeon*	*Yes, I agree. I cannot believe you've never had the chance to get trained in the use of this type of devices or drugs. No training, no optimal performance.*		
LEONARDO *Debriefer*	*I would like to ask you if you have ever experienced a similar situation in your clinical practice.*	•——►	The debriefer aims to link the reflection about actual events to previous experiences

Speaker	Dialogue		Comments
BEATRICE *Young* *anesthesiologist*	*The first time I had to replace the* *CO2 absorbant was a nightmare.* *And it was a regular surgery,* *fortunately. Not an emergency* *crisis, such as this we experienced* *here.*		
ARIANNA *Thoracic surgeon*	*We must inform the management.* *We must address the problem right* *now and find how to figure it out. A* *training session for the OR* *personnel could be the optimal* *option. We could use expired or* *about-to-expire drugs for the* *training. We could even save some* *money. I'm very happy this* *occurred in this simulation.*		
LEONARDO *Debriefer*	*"What we have to learn to do, we* *learn by doing it." Aristoteles* *already said this thousands of* *years ago.*	●→	The debriefer uses an aphorism to reinforce the effects of what has already been reached
ALL	*(Nodding)*		

Application Phase

Speaker	Dialogue		Comments
LEONARDO *Debriefer*	*Thank you all very much for this* *fruitful conversation. I think we* *have identified some very important* *elements which need rapid* *attention. Before leaving, I'd like to* *ask what are you taking home from* *this experience? What you would do* *next time you face a similar case?* *Try to think concretely, not* *generically. Something specific,* *truly feasible and achievable. Mark,* *would you like to start?*	●→	The debriefer invites each learner to share what they have learnt from the scenario and the debriefing. He encourages them to identify a SMART goal, thus the smallest actionable step, and dependent only on the learner, toward concrete and feasible change
MARK *Assistant* *surgeon*	*I have realized how important it is* *to share your thoughts with all the* *team, immediately, as soon as* *possible, I mean not only surgical* *team but with anesthesiologists,* *nurses, attendants, I mean everyone.*		

Speaker	Dialogue		Comments
LEONARDO *Debriefer*	*Thank you, Mark. So, to be practical, if in your next OR shift you experience a situation like the one we had today, what will you do?*	●→	Since the learner is too generic in the identification of his own goal, the debriefer facilitates the SMART one narrowing it to the next immediate time he'll encounter a similar situation. This is also for the benefit of the other learners who can understand better how to formulate a SMART goal, as requested by the debriefer
MARK *Assistant surgeon*	*Ok, next time, I'll ask for everyone's attention, and I'll rapidly report the emergency situation.*		
LEONARDO *Debriefer*	*Thank you, Mark. And you, Mary?*		
Mary	*Next time I bring something in the OR, I'll communicate that it has arrived and where I'm putting it directly to the person who ordered it. And I'll check he or she gets it.*		
(LEONARDO) (Debriefer)	*Very good. Beatrice, what will you do, then?*		
BEATRICE *Young anesthesiologist*	*Yes, probably I'll also call people directly by name, and I'll address to them personally the orders or requests. This is something I have to pay attention to.*		
LEONARDO *Debriefer*	*Thanks. And you Alessandra.*		
Alessandra	*My next shift is on next Friday, and I'll ask the head nurse to have the chance to learn how to prepare these blo***** complicated drugs! I was really scared, and I don't want to find myself in the same situation any more.*		
All	*(Nodding and laughing with her)*		
LEONARDO *Debriefer*	*(He turns and looks at Arianna)*		
ARIANNA *Thoracic surgeon*	*I think I will immediately call the head nurse to develop some training opportunities for our OR nursing personnel to avoid a situation like the one we just witnessed.*		

Speaker	Dialogue		Comments
LEONARDO *Debriefer*	*Thank you. That's very important. But you, what will you do personally if in your next intervention you experience an accidental vessel lesion?*	●—▶	The debriefer thanks Arianna for the valuable input. But he also stresses that Arianna should identify a personal goal
ARIANNA *Thoracic surgeon*	*Well, yes, I will check with the anesthesiologist about the priorities.*		
LEONARDO *Debriefer*	*Thank you very much, Arianna. And you, Sofia?*		
SOFIA *Scrub nurse*	*I'll also pay attention to whether the anesthesia team has been rapidly activated.*		
LEONARDO *Debriefer*	*Now it's my turn. At the beginning of my next shift, I'll check whether I remember the name of all my team members, and, in case not, I'll simply ask. Today's simulation has confirmed how important it is to activate people by calling them by name. It's known, in fact, that words have meaning and names have power.* *I sincerely thank you for your participation and your important input in this fruitful debriefing conversation.*	●—▶	Also, the debriefer shares what he has learned and his goal of change, in a circular learning situation. He closes with an echo effect to function as an anchor and emotional stabilization of one of the discovered elements cited by the learners